# HEART HEALTHY DIET AFTER 50

# Table of Contents

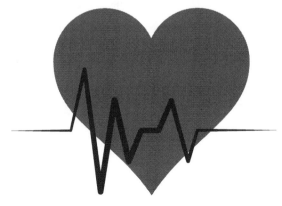

# INTRODUCTION

Welcome to "Heart Healthy Diet After 50." This cookbook is planned to help you embark on a journey towards healthier eating habits by providing you with a collection of delicious, nutritious recipes tailored for two people. In this introduction, we will explore the concept of healthy meals, the importance of incorporating them into your diet, tips for cooking nutritious meals, and the reasons to avoid fast food, canned and prepared meals, and sugary drinks.

What Are Healthy Meals?

Healthy meals are thoughtfully prepared using fresh, whole ingredients and designed to provide essential nutrients while maintaining a balanced diet. These meals typically include a variety of fruits, vegetables, lean proteins, whole grains, and healthy fats. They are low in added sugars, unhealthy fats, and excessive sodium.

## Why Should We Eat Healthy?

Eating healthy has numerous benefits for our overall well-being. A nutritious diet can contribute to maintaining a healthy weight, reducing the risk of chronic diseases such as heart disease, type 2 diabetes, and certain cancers. It supports proper digestion, boosts energy levels, enhances cognitive clarity, and strengthens the immune system. Moreover, healthy eating habits can improve mood, promote better sleep, and increase longevity.

## How to Cook Healthy Meals?

Cooking healthy meals doesn't have to be complicated or time-consuming. It starts with selecting fresh and wholesome ingredients. Opt for organic produce when possible, choose lean cuts of meat or plant-based proteins, incorporate whole grains like quinoa or brown rice, and use healthy oils such as olive or avocado oil for cooking. Balancing flavors with herbs, spices, and minimal amounts of salt can elevate the taste of your dishes while keeping the sodium content low. This cookbook will guide you through easy-to-follow recipes and provide valuable tips to help you create nutritious meals efficiently.

## Who Should Incorporate Healthy Food?

A healthy diet is beneficial for everyone, regardless of age or lifestyle. These recipes are designed for couples, ensuring portion control and minimizing food waste.

Whether you are a young couple starting a new chapter or simply someone who enjoys cooking, this cookbook will be an excellent resource for your culinary journey toward better health.

Why Avoid Fast Food, Canned, and Prepared Meals?

Fast food, canned, and prepared meals often contain excessive sodium, unhealthy fats, and added sugars. These foods are frequently linked to a higher risk of obesity, heart disease, high blood pressure, and other health issues. By avoiding these processed choices and instead focusing on homemade meals using fresh ingredients, you take control of your food's quality and nutritional value.

Why Not Drink Soda/Sugary Drinks?

Soda and other sugary drinks provide empty calories, offering little nutritional value. Habitually consuming these beverages has been associated with weight gain, increased risk of type 2 diabetes, tooth decay, and other adverse health effects. Instead, choose healthier drink choices such as water, unsweetened tea, herbal infusions, or naturally flavored water. These alternatives can keep you hydrated, support digestion, and contribute to overall well-being.

Benefits of a Healthy Diet

Embracing a healthy diet has numerous benefits. It can help you maintain a healthy weight, improve digestion, increase energy levels, enhance mental focus, and support a stronger immune system. Eating nutrient-dense foods can improve the appearance of your skin, hair, and nails while reducing the risk of chronic diseases. Additionally, a well-balanced diet can positively impact mood, promote restful sleep, and lead to a higher quality of life.

By incorporating the nutritious and flavorful recipes from this cookbook into your daily routine, you will embark on a path to better health, vitality, and culinary enjoyment.

## HEALTHY FATS:

1. Avocado and avocado oil
2. Olive oil
3. Coconut oil (in moderation)
4. Nuts and seeds (almonds, walnuts, chia seeds, flaxseeds)
5. Fatty fish (salmon, sardines, trout)
6. Nut butter (almond butter, peanut butter)
7. Full-fat dairy products (in moderation, for those who tolerate dairy)

## UNHEALTHY FATS to Limit or Avoid:

1. Trans fats (partially hydrogenated oils found in fried foods, packaged snacks, and some margarine)
2. Saturated fats (found in fatty cuts of meat and some processed foods)
3. Highly processed vegetable oils (corn oil, soybean oil, cottonseed oil)

## NATURAL SUGAR Substitutes:

1. Stevia
2. Monk fruit extract
3. Raw honey (in moderation)
4. Pure maple syrup (in moderation)
5. Dates or date paste
6. Unsweetened applesauce

## SALT SUBSTITUTES in Cooking:

1. Herbs and spices (such as garlic, onion powder, oregano, basil, turmeric, cumin, paprika)
2. Citrus juices (lemon, lime, orange) or zest
3. Vinegar (balsamic, apple cider, white wine)
4. Tamari or low-sodium soy sauce (use in moderation)
5. Homemade herb blends (combine dried herbs like thyme, rosemary, and parsley)

# HEAVY CREAM Alternatives:

Greek Yogurt is an excellent substitute for heavy cream in many dessert recipes. Its thick and creamy texture makes it perfect for dishes like puddings, cheesecakes, and mousses. Use an equal amount of Greek yogurt as a substitute.

Coconut Cream: Coconut cream is rich and creamy, making it an ideal substitute for heavy cream. It adds a subtle coconut flavor to the dish, which works well in tropical-themed desserts. Use the same amount of coconut cream as you would use heavy cream.

Silken Tofu: Silken tofu can be pureed and used as a substitute for heavy cream in recipes like creamy pies, custards, and mousse. It adds a smooth and silky texture to the dish while reducing the calorie content significantly.

Cashew Cream: Soak raw cashews overnight, drain them, and blend them with a small quantity of water until smooth to create cashew cream. This cream is similar in consistency to heavy cream and works well in sauces, frostings, and creamy desserts.

Evaporated Milk: Evaporated milk is a lighter, lower-fat alternative to heavy cream. It works well in recipes that require thickening, such as custards, sauces, and pies. Substitute an equal amount of evaporated milk for heavy cream.

Almond Milk or Oat Milk: Unsweetened almond or oat milk can be used in recipes requiring heavy cream, especially baked ones like cakes and muffins. However, remember that the texture may not be as rich or creamy as other substitutes. Use an equal amount of almond milk or oat milk.

Cottage Cheese: In some dessert recipes, such as cheesecakes or fruit parfaits, you can replace heavy cream with blended cottage cheese. This substitution adds protein and reduces the fat content.

If the recipe calls for whipping heavy cream, some alternatives may whip to a different extent. To improve consistency, you can try chilling the substitute in the refrigerator before beating it.

Be mindful that flavor and texture may vary when substituting heavy cream, but the overall result can still be delicious.

# NATURALLY FLAVORED WATER

You can use various ingredients that add a refreshing taste without relying on artificial additives or excessive sugar. Here's a list of ingredients you can use and some tips to make naturally flavored water:

Citrus Fruits: Slice lemons, limes, oranges, or grapefruits and add them to your water. Citrus fruits provide a burst of flavor and are rich in vitamin C.

Berries: Raspberries, strawberries, blueberries, or blackberries are great choices. Crush the berries slightly to release their flavors.

Cucumber and Mint: Slice a cucumber and add a few sprigs of fresh mint. This combination is both refreshing and hydrating.

Watermelon: Cut fresh watermelon into cubes or use a melon baller. Watermelon contains high water content and adds a sweet, juicy taste.

Herbs: Experiment with herbs like basil, rosemary, or lavender. These herbs infuse water with subtle, aromatic flavors.

Ginger: Grate or slice fresh ginger to add a zing to your water. Ginger has a cleansing effect and can aid digestion.

Citrus Zest: Use a zester to add small amounts of zest from citrus fruits like lemon, lime, or orange. The zest contains essential oils that provide a burst of flavor.

Cinnamon Sticks: Add a cinnamon stick to your water for a hint of warm and sweet flavor. Cinnamon is known for its antioxidant properties.

Hibiscus Flowers: Dried hibiscus flowers create a vibrant red drink with a tart and tangy taste. Steep the flowers in cold water for a few hours.

Fruit Infuser: Invest in a fruit infuser bottle or pitcher. These allow you to place fruits and herbs inside a separate compartment, infusing their flavors into the water without any residue.

Tips for preparing naturally flavored water:

1. Wash all fruits and herbs thoroughly before using them.
2. Cut the ingredients into small pieces or crush them slightly to release their flavors.
3. For a stronger flavor, gently muddle the fruits and herbs before adding them to the water.
4. Use filtered or purified water to enhance the taste.
5. Let the water infuse for at least an hour in the refrigerator to allow the flavors to meld together. The longer you infuse, the stronger the flavor.
6. Experiment with different combinations and adjust the ingredient quantities according to your taste preferences.

Naturally flavored water might not taste as sweet as artificially flavored drinks, but it offers a healthier and more refreshing alternative.

## NATURAL VEGETABLE STOCK

Ingredients:
- 2 onions, roughly chopped
- 2 carrots, roughly chopped
- 2 celery stalks, roughly chopped
- 2 garlic cloves, minced
- 1 leek, white and light green parts only, roughly chopped
- 1 parsnip, roughly chopped
- 1 turnip, roughly chopped
- 1 handful of fresh parsley
- 2 bay leaves
- 1 teaspoon whole peppercorns
- 8 cups of water
- Salt, to taste

Instructions:
Heat a large pot over medium heat and add a splash of water (or a small amount of olive oil if preferred). Add the onions, carrots, celery, leek, garlic, parsnip, and turnip. Sauté the vegetables for about 5 minutes, stirring occasionally, until they start to soften. Add the parsley, bay leaves, and peppercorns to the pot. Stir well to combine. Pour in the water, ensuring that the vegetables are completely covered. Increase the heat to high and bring the mixture to a boil.

Once the stock reaches a boil, reduce the heat to low and let it simmer uncovered for about 45 minutes to 1 hour. This allows the flavors to meld together and the vegetables to release their essence. After simmering, remove the pot from the heat and let it cool slightly. Strain the stock into another pot or a large bowl using a fine-mesh sieve or a cheesecloth-lined colander. Press down on the vegetables to extract as much liquid as possible. Discard the solids, or use a hand mixer to mix the vegetable and leave them in the water. Taste the stock and add salt as needed, depending on your preference. Let the stock cool completely before storing it. Once cooled, transfer it to airtight containers or freeze it in ice cube trays for easy portioning.

Note: You can customize this recipe by adding or substituting other vegetables like mushrooms, bell peppers, or fennel, depending on your taste preferences and what you have available.

There are several reasons why making vegetable stock using a homemade recipe is beneficial compared to using store-bought, like beef or chicken stock:

Healthier Option:
The vegetable stock is an excellent choice for vegetarians, vegans, or those looking to reduce their consumption of animal products. It provides a flavorful base for various dishes without using animal-derived ingredients.

Lower Sodium Content:
Store-bought stocks, particularly those made from meat, often contain high sodium levels to enhance the flavor.

By making your vegetable stock, you control the amount of salt added, making it a healthier option, especially for individuals monitoring their sodium intake.

Control over Ingredients:
Making vegetable stock at home allows you to choose the quality of the ingredients and ensure there are no additives, preservatives, or artificial flavors. It allows you to use fresh, organic vegetables and customize the flavor.

Versatility:
The vegetable stock has a neutral flavor profile, making it a versatile base for various recipes. It can be used in soups, stews, sauces, risotto, and other dishes, providing a subtle and complementary flavor without overpowering the other ingredients.

Nutrient-Rich:
Homemade vegetable stock retains the nutrients in the vegetables, such as vitamins, minerals, and antioxidants. These nutrients contribute to the overall nutritional value of the dishes you prepare using the stock.

Cost-Effective:
Making your vegetable stock can be more cost-effective than buying pre-packaged stocks. It allows you to use leftover vegetable scraps or parts that would otherwise be discarded, reducing waste and saving money.

Customizable Flavors:

With homemade vegetable stock, you can adjust the flavors to your liking. You can experiment with different combinations of vegetables and herbs, tailoring the stock to match your preferences and the specific dish you're preparing.

While store-bought stocks can be convenient, making your vegetable stock offers numerous benefits regarding taste, nutrition, and control over ingredients. It's a simple and rewarding process that allows you to create a flavorful and healthy foundation for your culinary creations.

# MAYONNAISE ALTERNATIVES

Mayonnaise is a popular condiment but can be high in calories and unhealthy fats. Here are some options:

Greek Yogurt: Greek yogurt is a versatile and nutritious substitute for mayonnaise. It has a creamy texture and tangy flavor and works well in dressings, dips, and spreads. You can use it as a 1:1 replacement for mayonnaise in most recipes.

Avocado: Mashed avocado can be a delicious and creamy alternative to mayonnaise. It adds healthy fats and provides a smooth texture. Use ripe avocado as a spread or mix it into salads and dressings for a creamy consistency.

Hummus: Hummus is made from blended chickpeas, tahini, and other ingredients. It has a creamy texture and offers a flavorful substitute for mayonnaise.

You can use hummus as a spread on sandwiches or wraps or as a vegetable dip.

Mustard: Mustard is a low-calorie and flavorful alternative to mayonnaise. It adds a tangy taste to sandwiches, wraps, and salad dressings. Choose your favorite types of mustard, such as Dijon or whole grain, to suit your preferences.

Nut or Seed Butter: Nuts or seed butter, such as almond butter or tahini, can be used as a healthy alternative to mayonnaise. They provide richness and creaminess to recipes while adding nutrients and healthy fats. Adjust the amount based on your desired consistency and flavor.

Greek Yogurt-Based Dressings: Many brands offer Greek yogurt-based dressings that mimic the creamy texture of mayonnaise-based sauces. Look for options like Greek yogurt ranch or Caesar dressings, which can be used in salads or as dips.

Vinaigrettes: Light and tangy vinaigrettes made with olive oil, vinegar, and herbs can provide a healthy alternative to creamy dressings. They add flavor and moisture to salads without the high-calorie content of mayonnaise.

You can experiment with these alternatives and adjust the seasonings and flavors to suit your preferences. Some recipes are in this cookbook. Please consider the specific recipe or dish you're preparing to ensure the substitute complements the other ingredients.

# Conclusion

You can modify the ingredients of any recipe in this cookbook using the healthy tips provided in the introduction. You can begin a journey of culinary experimentation to discover what suits your preferences and aligns with your personal health goals. With minor changes to the ingredients used in recipes, you can enhance the nutritional value of your meals without compromising on taste.

One suggestion mentioned in the introduction is to replace salt with different spices. Salt is commonly used to enhance flavors in cooking, but excessive sodium consumption can negatively affect our health. By substituting salt with various spices, such as garlic powder, paprika, cumin, or turmeric, we not only add depth and complexity to our dishes but also benefit from these spices' unique health properties and flavors.
Additionally, herbs like rosemary, thyme, or basil can provide freshness and aroma to your meals.

Another recommendation is to replace sugar with stevia, a natural and zero-calorie sweetener derived from the stevia plant. While sugar adds sweetness to recipes, excessive sugar intake has been linked to various health concerns. Stevia can be a suitable alternative, as it provides sweetness without the added calories and potential negative effects associated with refined sugar. When using stevia, it's important to note that it is significantly sweeter than sugar, so you'll need less of it to achieve the desired level of sweetness.

# MEASUREMENTS

Now, let's talk about the approximate measurements provided in the cookbook. These measurements can be a helpful guideline when preparing recipes, ensuring your culinary creations turn out as intended. It's important to note that these measurements are approximate and may vary slightly depending on factors such as the density of the ingredient or the specific conversion standards used in different regions.

The cookbook suggests that 1 cup is roughly equivalent to 250 grams or 8.8 ounces for liquid ingredients. This measurement can help you accurately portion your recipes' liquids like water, milk, or broth.

Regarding sugar, the suggested conversion is 1 cup to approximately 200 grams or 7.0 ounces. This measurement is convenient if you want to reduce the amount of sugar in a recipe or substitute it with an alternative sweetener like stevia or sweetener.

Lastly, the cookbook recommends that 1 cup corresponds to around 120 grams or 4.8 ounces of flour. This approximation allows you to precisely measure flour for baking or cooking purposes, ensuring the right consistency and texture in your final dish.

# BREAKFAST

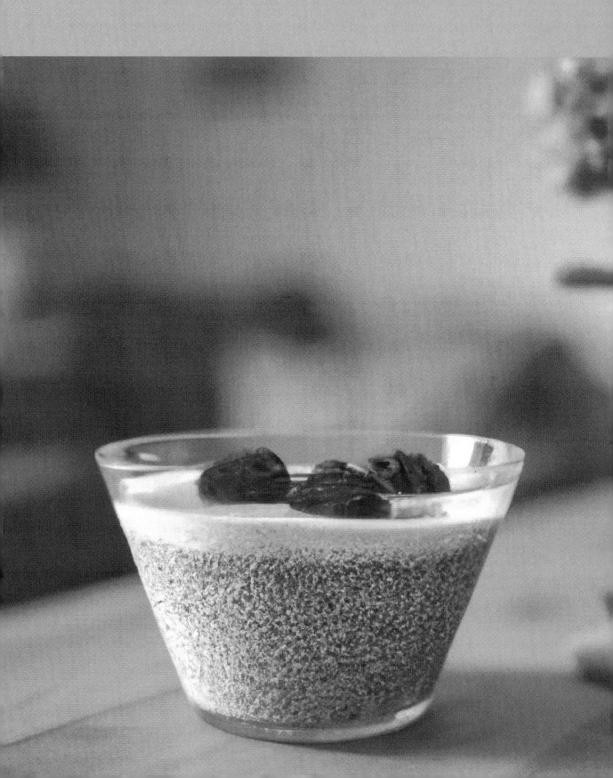

# Coconut Yogurt

Servings: 2          Prep time: 2 hours          Cook time: 10 min

## INGREDIENTS

1 probiotic capsule - yogurt capsule
1 cup of coconut milk
1 tbsp of coconut meat
4 tbsps of chia seeds

Nutrition:
- Calories: 583
- Fat: 46.9 g
- Fiber: 22.9g
- Carbs: 36g
- Protein: 12.6g
- Cholesterol 0mg
- Sodium 35mg

## DIRECTIONS

Pour coconut milk into the saucepan, and preheat it to 108F/42C. Then add a probiotic capsule and stir well. Close the lid and leave the coconut milk for 40 minutes. Meanwhile, shred coconut meat. When it is over, squeeze the milk mixture into the cheesecloth. Leave it for 40 minutes or until the yogurt's liquid is squeezed. After this, transfer the yogurt into the serving glasses. Add chia seeds and coconut meat in every glass and mix up well. Let the cooked yogurt rest for 10 minutes before serving.

# Shrimp Skillet

Servings: 2          Prep time: 15 min          Cook time: 25min

## INGREDIENTS

2 bell peppers
1 red onion
1-pound of shrimps, peeled
½ tsp of white pepper
½ tsp of paprika
1 tbsp of olive oil

Nutrition:
- Calories: 153
- Fat: 4 g
- Fiber: 1.3 g
- Carbs: 7.3 g
- Protein: 21.5 g
- Cholesterol 197 mg
- Potassium 284 mg

## DIRECTIONS

Remove the seeds from the bell peppers and, cut the vegetable into wedges, place them in the skillet. Add peeled shrimp, white pepper, paprika, and oil. Peel and slice the red onion. Add it to the skillet too. Preheat the oven to 365F/185C. Cover the skillet with foil and secure the edges. Transfer it to the preheated oven and cook for 20 minutes. When the time is over, discard the foil and cook the dish for 5 minutes more. Use ventilation mode if you have one.

# Egg Fat Bombs

Servings: 2          Prep time: 20 min          Cook time: 10 min

INGREDIENTS

4 oz. of bacon, sliced

4 eggs, boiled

salt

½ tsp of ground

black pepper

1 tbsp of mayonnaise

Nutrition:
- Calories: 463
- Fat: 34.3 g
- Fiber: 0.1 g
- Carbs: 3.6 g
- Protein: 32.1 g
- Cholesterol: 392 mg
- Sodium: 2067mg

DIRECTIONS

Line the tray with baking paper. Place the bacon on the form. Preheat the oven to 365F/185C and put the tray inside. Cook the bacon for 10 minutes or until it is light brown. Meanwhile, peel and chop the boiled eggs and transfer them to the mixing bowl. Add the ground black pepper, mayonnaise, and salt. Chill it a little when the bacon is cooked, and finely chop it. Add the bacon to the egg mixture, and stir it well. With the help of the scoop, make medium size balls. Before serving, place them in the fridge for 10 minutes.

# Chia Pudding

Servings: 2          Prep time: 15 min          Cook time: 3min

INGREDIENTS

2 cups of almond milk

8 tbsps of chia seeds

1 oz. of blackberries

1 tbsp of Erythritol or stevia

DIRECTIONS

Preheat the almond milk for 3 minutes; remove it from the heat and add chia seeds. Stir gently and add the Erythritol. Mix it up. In the bottom of the serving glasses, put the blackberries. Then pour the almond milk mixture over the berries. Let the pudding rest for at least 10 minutes before serving.

Nutrition:
- Calories: 580
- Fat: 57.9 g
- Fiber: 10.7 g
- Carbs: 16.8 g
- Protein: 5.6 g
- Cholesterol: 0
- Sodium: 36 mg

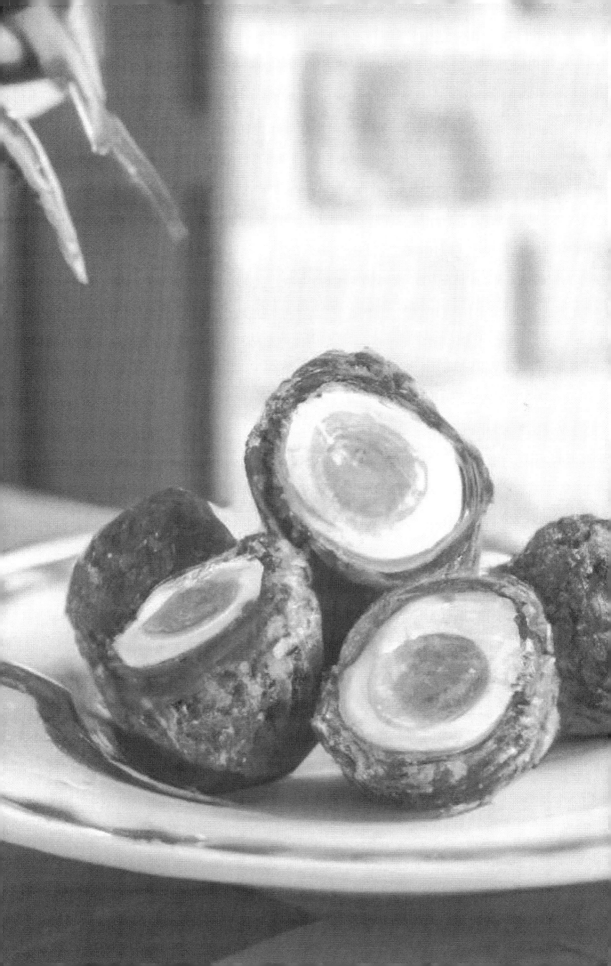

# Scotch Eggs

Servings: 2          Prep time: 15 min          Cook time: 15 min

## INGREDIENTS

4 eggs, boiled
1 ½ cup of ground beef
1 tbsp of onion, grated
½ tsp of ground
black pepper
salt
½ tsp of dried oregano
½ tsp of dried basil
1 tbsp of olive oil
¾ cup of water

Nutrition:
- Calories: 498
- Fat: 25.4 g
- Fiber: 0.2 g
- Carbs: 1.7 g
- Protein: 62.9 g
- Cholesterol: 495 mg
- Sodium: 861 mg

## DIRECTIONS

Mix the ground beef, grated onion, black pepper, salt, dried oregano, and basil in the bowl. Peel the boiled eggs. Make 4 balls from the ground beef mixture. Put peeled eggs inside every ground beef ball and press them gently to get the shape of the eggs. Spread the tray with the oil and place ground beef eggs on it. Add water. Preheat the oven to 365F/185C and transfer the tray inside. Cook the dish for 15 minutes or until each side of Scotch eggs is light brown.

# Bacon Pancakes

Servings: 2          Prep time: 10 min          Cook time: 25 min

## INGREDIENTS

3 oz. of bacon, chopped
½ cup of almond flour
¾ cup of light cream
½ tsp of baking powder
salt
1 egg, whisked

Nutrition:
- Calories: 448
- Fat: 36.4 g
- Fiber: 0.2 g
- Carbs: 3.6 g
- Protein: 40.9 g
- Cholesterol: 190 mg
- Sodium: 1322mg

## DIRECTIONS

Place the chopped bacon in the skillet and cook it for 5-6 minutes over medium-high heat. The cooked bacon should be crunchy. Meanwhile, mix up the almond flour, light cream, salt, baking powder, and whisked egg. When the mixture is smooth, the batter is cooked. Add the cooked bacon to the batter and stir it gently with the help of the spoon. Don't clean the skillet after the bacon. Ladle the bacon batter in the skillet and make the pancake. Cook it for 1 minute from one side and then flip it onto another. Cook it for 2 minutes more. Make the same steps with the remaining batter. Transfer the pancakes to the serving plate.

# Mediterranean Omelette

Servings: 2          Prep time: 20 min          Cook time: 10 min

INGREDIENTS

3 eggs, beaten
1 tbsp of ricotta cheese
2 oz. of feta cheese, chopped
1 tomato, chopped
1 tsp of olive oil
salt
1 tbsp of scallions, chopped

DIRECTIONS

Mix up the ricotta cheese and eggs. Add salt and scallions. Toss the oil in the skillet and melt it. Pour ½ part of the whisked egg mixture into the skillet and cook it for 5-6 minutes or until it is solid—the omelet is cooked. Then transfer the omelet to the plate. Make the second omelet with the remaining egg mixture. Sprinkle each omelet with Feta and tomatoes. Roll them.

Nutrition:
- Calories: 205
- Fat: 15.9 g
- Fiber: 3.9 g
- Carbs: 3.5 g
- Protein: 13.6 g
- Cholesterol: 278 mg
- Sodium: 1015 mg

# Avocado Toast

Servings: 2          Prep time: 10 min          Cook time: 4min

INGREDIENTS

2 small avocado, ripe
4 slices bread, of choice
1 garlic clove
extra virgin olive oil
lemon juice
cilantro finely chopped

DIRECTIONS

Toast the bread to taste. Cut the avocado in half, and remove the seed. Lightly rub the toasted bread's surface with the garlic clove's cut side. Use a spoon to scoop the avocado flesh out, then a fork to mush it onto the toast. Squeeze over some lemon juice, drizzle with olive oil, then sprinkle with cilantro.

Nutrition:
- Calories: 526
- Fat: 46.8 g
- Fiber: 14.4g
- Carbs: 28g
- Protein: 5.8g
- Cholesterol: 0mg
- Sodium: 148mg

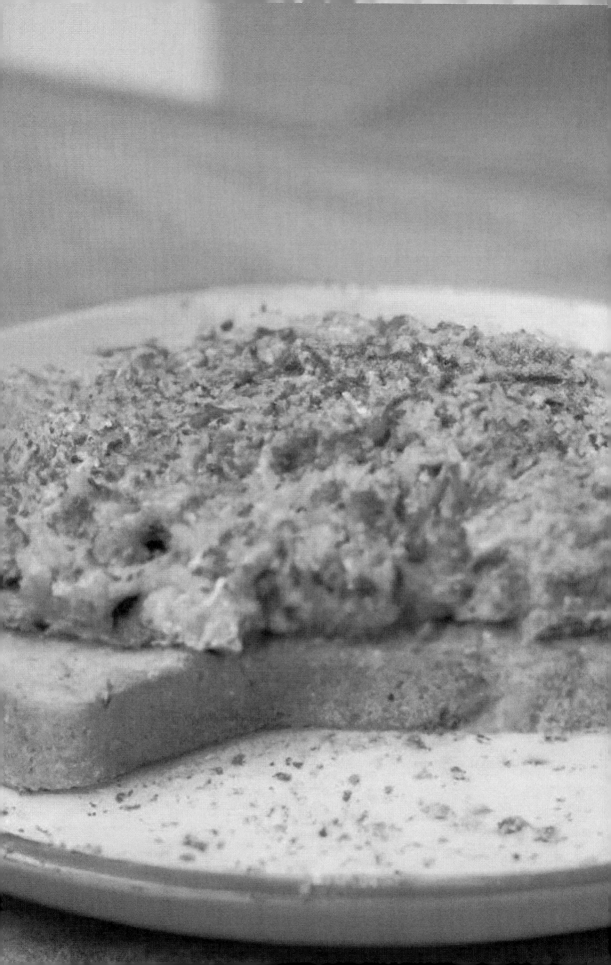

# Matcha Fat Bombs

Servings: 2        Prep time: 15 min        Cook time: 0 min

## INGREDIENTS

½ cup of cashew butter

1 cup of coconut butter

¼ cup of coconut cream

2 tbsps of matcha green tea

¼ tsp of ground cinnamon

½ cup of coconut shred

Nutrition:
- Calories: 923
- Fat: 74.6g
- Fiber: 11.1g
- Carbs: 32.5g
- Protein: 10.5g
- Cholesterol: 0mg
- Sodium: 48mg

## DIRECTIONS

Put the cashew butter, coconut butter, coconut cream, ½ tbsp of matcha green tea, and ground cinnamon in the mixing bowl. Blend the mixture with the hand blender until you get a homogenous and fluffy mass. Mix the coconut shred and remaining matcha green tea in a separate bowl. Make the balls from the coconut butter mixture with the help of the scooper. Then coat every ball in the coconut shred green mixture. Transfer the meal to the plates and store them in the fridge.

# Cinnamon Toast

Servings: 2        Prep time: 10min        Cook time: 5min

## INGREDIENTS

4 bread slices

2 tbsp unsalted butter

2 tbsps of stevia

2 tsp of ground cinnamon

½ tsp of vanilla extract

Nutrition:
- Calories: 158
- Fat: 12.3 g
- Fiber: 1.7 g
- Carbs: 11.1 g
- Protein: 1.6 g
- Cholesterol: 31mg
- Sodium: 205 mg

## DIRECTIONS

Combine the butter, cinnamon, stevia, and vanilla extract in a bowl. Spread onto the slices of bread. Set your Air Fryer to 380F/180C. When warmed up, put the bread inside the fryer and cook for 4– 5 minutes, or use the oven for 7 min at 392F/200C.

# Hash Brown

## INGREDIENTS

12 oz. of grated fresh cauliflower -about ½ a medium-sized head
4 slices of bacon, chopped
3 oz. of onion, chopped
1 tbsp of butter, softened

## DIRECTIONS

In a skillet, sauté the bacon and onion until brown. Add in the cauliflower and stir until tender and browned. Add the butter steadily as it cooks. Season to taste with salt and pepper.

Nutrition:
- Calories: 307
- Fat: 21.8g
- Fiber: 4.2g
- Carbs: 11.5g
- Protein: 17.2g
- Cholesterol: 57mg
- Sodium: 960mg

# Vegetable Toast

## INGREDIENTS

4 slices of bread
1 red bell pepper, cut into strips
1 cup of a sliced button or cremini mushrooms
1 small yellow squash, sliced
2 green onions, sliced
1 tbsp of olive oil
2 tbsps of softened butter
½ cup of soft goat cheese

## DIRECTIONS

Drizzle the Air Fryer with olive oil and preheat to 350F/176C. Put the red pepper, green onions, mushrooms, and squash inside the fryer, stir them, and cook for 7 minutes, shaking the basket once throughout the cooking time. Ensure the vegetables become tender. Remove the vegetables and set them aside. Spread some butter on the slices of bread and transfer to the Air Fryer, butter side-up. Brown for 2 to 4 minutes. Remove the toast from the fryer and top it with goat cheese and vegetables. Serve warm.

Nutrition:
- Calories: 253
- Fat: 19.3 g
- Fiber: 2.5 g
- Carbs: 18.2 g
- Protein: 4 g
- Cholesterol: 31mg
- Sodium: 137 mg

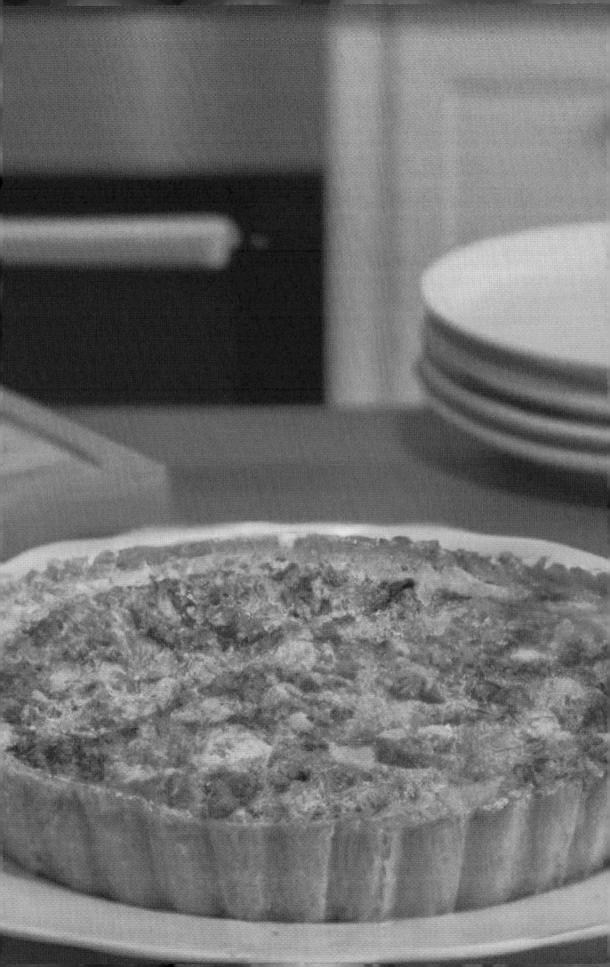

# Noatmeal

Servings: 2          Prep time: 10min          Cook time: 10 min

## INGREDIENTS

1 cup of organic almond milk
2 tbsps of hemp seeds
1 tbsp of chia seeds, dried
1 tbsp of Erythritol
1 tbsp of almond flakes
2 tbsps of coconut flour
1 tbsp of flax meal
1 tbsp of walnuts, chopped
½ tsp of vanilla extract
¼ tsp of ground cinnamon

Nutrition:
- Calories: 350
- Fat: 30.4 g
- Fiber: 8.4 g
- Carbs: 16.9 g
- Protein: 9.1 g
- Cholesterol: 358mg
- Sodium: 18 mg

## DIRECTIONS

Put all the ingredients except vanilla extract in the saucepan and stir gently. Cook the mixture on low heat for 10 minutes. Stir it constantly. When the mixture starts to be thick, add vanilla extract. Mix it up. Remove the oatmeal from the heat and let it rest a little.

# Feta Quiche

Servings: 2          Prep time: 15min          Cook time: 30min

## INGREDIENTS

8 oz. of Feta cheese,
5 eggs, whisked
1 cup of spinach, chopped
1 garlic clove, diced
1 white onion, diced
1 tsp of olive oil
5 oz. of Mozzarella, chopped
½ tsp of chili flakes
1 tsp of paprika
½ tsp of white pepper
½ cup of whipped light cream

Nutrition:
- Calories: 350
- Fat: 59.4 g
- Fiber: 2.1 g
- Carbs: 16.8 g
- Protein: 52.1 g
- Cholesterol: 358mg
- Sodium: 1888 mg

## DIRECTIONS

Heat oil in the skillet, add the diced garlic and onion, and cook it over medium heat until soft. Transfer to the mixing bowl. Add the crumbled cheese, whisked eggs, spinach, chopped Mozzarella, chili flakes, paprika, white pepper, and whipped cream to the bowl. Combine the mixture well and transfer it to the non-sticky mold. Flatten it gently with the spatula. Place the mold in the preheated 365F/185C oven and cook the quiche for 25 minutes. Chill the quiche a little and then cut it into servings.

# Waffles

Servings: 2          Prep time: 10min          Cook time: 15 min

## INGREDIENTS

2 tbsps of olive oil, melted
4 eggs, whisked
1 tsp of baking powder
1 tsp of lemon juice
1 cup of almond flour
½ tsp of vanilla extract
1 tbsp of Erythritol
¾ cup of organic almond milk

## DIRECTIONS

In the mixing bowl, combine all the ingredients. Whisk the smooth and homogenous batter. Preheat the waffle maker well. Pour enough of the oil into the waffle maker. Flatten it gently to get a waffle. Close it and cook until lightly golden. Repeat the same steps with all remaining batter. Serve the waffles warm.

Nutrition:
- Calories: 442
- Fat: 41 g
- Fiber: 37 g
- Carbs: 8 g
- Protein: 13.6 g
- Cholesterol: 358 mg
- Sodium: 221 mg

# Spinach Egg

Servings: 2          Prep time: 10min          Cook time: 30min

## INGREDIENTS

3 whole eggs
3 oz. of cottage cheese
3-4 oz. of chopped spinach
¼ cup of parmesan cheese
¼ cup of milk

## DIRECTIONS

Preheat your oven to 375F/190C. Whisk the eggs, cottage cheese, parmesan, and milk in a large bowl. Mix in the spinach. Transfer to a small, greased oven dish. Sprinkle the cheese on top. Bake for 25-30 minutes. Let it cool for 5 minutes and serve.

Nutrition:
- Calories:172
- Fat: 9 g
- Fiber: 1.3 g
- Carbs: 5.7 g
- Protein: 17.9 g
- Cholesterol: 254 mg
- Sodium: 357 mg

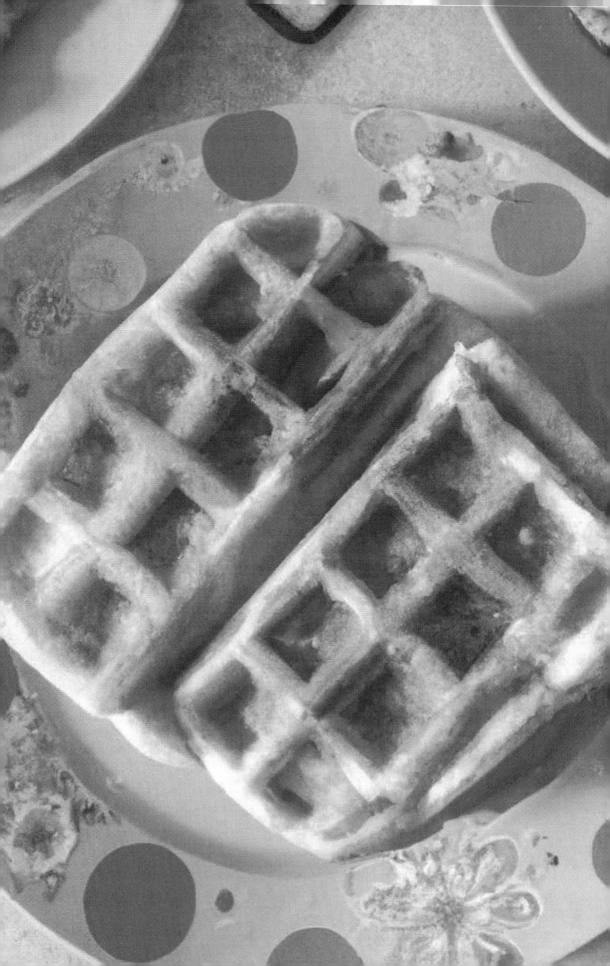

# Omelette

Servings: 2          Prep time: 10min          Cook time: 20 min

### INGREDIENTS

1 cup of mushrooms, chopped
½ white onion, sliced
½ tsp of tomato paste
2 tbsps of water
½ tsp of salt
½ tsp of cayenne pepper
¾ tsp of chili flakes
3 eggs, beaten
1 tbsp of cream cheese
1 tsp of butter
1 tsp of avocado oil

Nutrition:
- Calories: 152
- Fat: 10.7 g
- Fiber: 1.2 g
- Carbs: 5 g
- Protein: 10.3 g
- Cholesterol: 256 mg
- Sodium: 707 mg

### DIRECTIONS

Pour the avocado oil into the skillet and preheat it. Add the chopped mushrooms and sliced onion. Then add the tomato paste and water. Stir the ingredients and sauté them with the closed lid for 10 minutes. Transfer the cooked vegetables to the mixing bowl. Whisk the cream cheese, eggs, chili flakes, cayenne pepper, and salt. Toss the butter in the skillet and melt it. Add the egg mixture. Close the lid. Cook it for 10 minutes over medium-low heat. Then spread the mushroom mixture over the cooked omelet and roll it. Cut the cooked meal into 2 parts and transfer it to the serving plates.

# Zucchini Bread

Servings: 2          Prep time: 15 min          Cook time: 50min

### INGREDIENTS

½ cup of walnuts, chopped
1 tsp of baking powder
1 tbsp of lemon juice
1 tbsp of flax meal
1 ½ cup of almond flour
1 zucchini, grated
1 tsp of xanthan gum
1 tbsp of butter, melted
3 eggs, beaten
salt

Nutrition:
- Calories: 390
- Fat: 32.2 g
- Fiber: 4.3 g
- Carbs: 9.2 g
- Protein: 17.9 g
- Cholesterol: 261 mg
- Sodium: 1310 mg

### DIRECTIONS

Preheat oven to 360F/180C. In the mixing bowl, combine all wet ingredients. Whisk the mixture well. Then add baking powder, flax meal, almond flour, zucchini, xanthan gum, and salt. Combine the mixture. Add chopped walnuts and stir it well. You will get a liquid but thick dough. Transfer the dough to the non-sticky loaf mold and flatten its surface with the spatula. Place the bread in the oven and cook for 50 minutes. Check if the bread is cooked with the help of the toothpick —if it is clean—the bread is cooked. Remove the zucchini bread from the oven and chill well, then remove it from the mold and let it cool.

# Granola

Servings: 2          Prep time: 10min          Cook time: 25 min

## INGREDIENTS

4 tbsps of walnuts
3 tbsps of pecans
3 tbsps of hazelnuts
1 tbsp of chia seeds
2 tbsps of pumpkin seeds
2 tbsps of flax meal
1 tbsp of coconut shred
1 tbsp of Erythritol
2 tbsps of almond butter
1 tbsp of peanut butter

Nutrition:
- Calories: 152
- Fat: 10.7 g
- Fiber: 1.2 g
- Carbs: 5 g
- Protein: 10.3 g
- Cholesterol: 256 mg
- Sodium: 707 mg

## DIRECTIONS

Chop the walnuts, pecans, hazelnuts, and pumpkin seeds, and transfer them to the mixing bowl. Add the chia seeds, flax meal, coconut shred, Erythritol, almond butter, and peanut butter. Blend the mixture. The mass should be sticky. Preheat the oven to 300F/150C. Line the tray with parchment. Transfer the nut mixture to the parchment and flatten it into the layer. Place the tray in the oven and cook it for 25 minutes. When the time is over, remove the tray from the oven and chill the granola. Cut it into medium size pieces. Store granola in a glass jar with a closed lid.

# Cheese Souffle

Servings: 2          Prep time: 25 min          Cook time: 15 min

## INGREDIENTS

2 oz. of Cheddar cheese, grated
½ tsp of ground black pepper
½ tsp of salt
½ cup of almond milk
½ onion
1 bay leaf
¼ tsp of peppercorn
1 tbsp of coconut shred
2 tsp of butter, melted
2 eggs
1 tsp of coconut oil
2 cups of almond flour
½ tsp of paprika

## DIRECTIONS

Brush the ramekins with coconut oil and sprinkle with coconut shreds. Then pour ¼ cup of the almond milk into the saucepan. Add onion and peppercorns. Bring it to a boil. Remove the onion and peppercorns. Toss the butter in the pan and add the almond flour. Stir it well until smooth. Add the salt, ground black pepper, and paprika. Mix up well. After this, separate the egg yolk and egg whites. Add the egg yolks to the almond flour mixture, and stir it well. Add the other ¼ cup of almond milk and start to preheat it. Stir it all the time until the mixture is smooth. Whisk the egg whites until they have firm peaks.

See next page                    34

# Cheese Soufle

Servings: 2          Prep time: min          Cook time: min

## INGREDIENTS

## DIRECTIONS

Continue from the previous page:
Add the grated Cheddar to the almond flour mixture. Mix it up. Then chill the mixture a little. Add the egg whites and mix gently—Preheat the oven to 365F/185C. Place the cheese mixture into the prepared ramekins and transfer it to the tray. Put the tray in the preheated oven and cook for 15 minutes. When the soufflé is cooked, it will have a light brown color.

Nutrition:
- Calories:390
- Fat: 34.2 g
- Fiber: 2.3 g
- Carbs: 7.2 g
- Protein: 14.5 g
- Cholesterol: 204 mg
- Sodium: 857 mg

# Oat Muffins

Servings: 2          Prep time: 15 min          Cook time: 35min

## INGREDIENTS

1 1/2 cups smashed very ripe bananas
2 large eggs
2 cups rolled oats, plus more for topping
¼ cup sunflower oil
¼ cup pure maple syrup
1 tbsp vanilla extract
1 tsp baking powder
1 tsp cinnamon

Nutrition:
- Calories: 931
- Fat: 38.2 g
- Fiber: 14.2 g
- Carbs: 131.8 g
- Protein: 19.3 g
- Cholesterol: 186 mg
- Sodium: 161 mg

## DIRECTIONS

Preheat the oven to 350F/176C. Place all ingredients in a blender, and blend everything on high until a smooth batter forms. Place muffin cups into a muffin tin and pour the batter divided evenly between the cups. Sprinkle the tops with extra oats and gently press them down. Bake for about 30 to 35 minutes until a toothpick comes out clean. Remove from the muffin tin and allow them to cool a few minutes before serving.

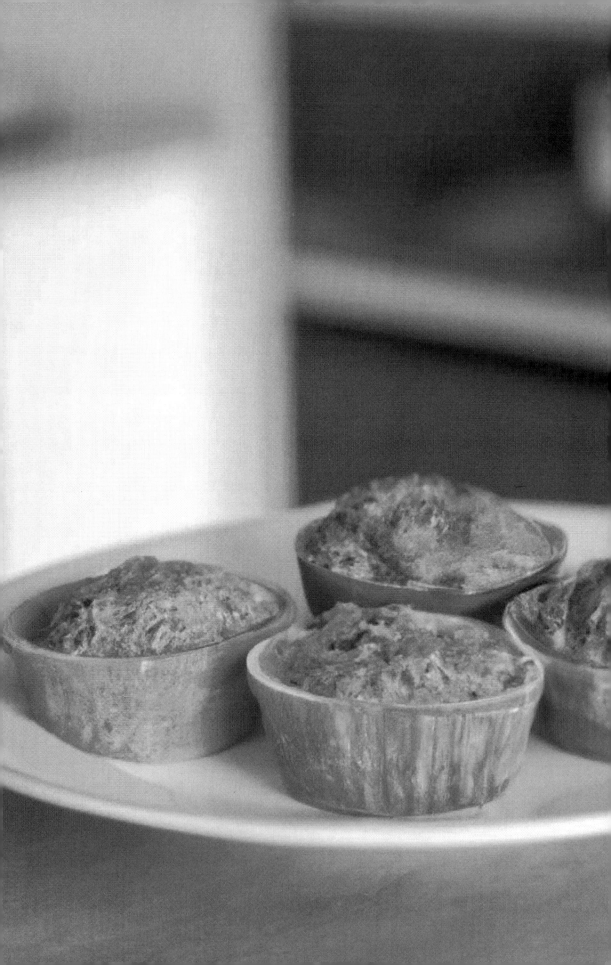

# Easy Blended Pancakes

Servings: 2          Prep time: 15min          Cook time: 5min

## INGREDIENTS

2 eggs
2 oz. of cream cheese
1 scoop Isopure Protein Powder or any
1 pinch of salt
1 dash of cinnamon

## DIRECTIONS

Mix the eggs with cream cheese, protein powder, salt, and cinnamon in a bowl. Transfer to a blender and blend until smooth. Heat a nonstick pan and pour a quarter of the mixture. Cook for about 2 minutes on each side and dish out. Repeat with the remaining mix and dish out on a platter to serve warm.

Nutrition:
- Calories: 222
- Fat: 15.2 g
- Fiber: 0.1 g
- Carbs: 3.1 g
- Protein: 18.8 g
- Cholesterol: 227 mg
- Sodium: 251 mg

# Chicken Fritters

Servings: 2          Prep time: 10 min          Cook time: 8min

## INGREDIENTS

1-pound of chicken fillet, finely chopped
2 tbsps of almond flour
1 egg, beaten
1 tsp of dried dill
1 tsp of dried oregano
salt
1 tsp of minced garlic
1 tbsp of olive oil

## DIRECTIONS

Put the finely chopped chicken fillet and almond flour in the mixing bowl. Add beaten egg, dried dill, oregano, salt, and minced garlic. Mix it up. Make the fritters. Pour olive oil into the skillet and preheat it until hot. Add the fritters and fry them for 4 minutes from each side over medium heat. Dry the fritters with the help of a paper towel and transfer them to the serving bowl.

Nutrition:
- Calories: 528
- Fat: 26.7 g
- Carbs: 1.4 g
- Protein: 68,7 g
- Cholesterol:  284 mg
- Sodium: 809 mg

# Eggs Portobello Mushroom

Servings: 2          Prep time: 10min          Cook time: 15 min

INGREDIENTS

4 Portobello caps
4 quail eggs
½ tsp of dried parsley
salt
1 tsp of butter, melted

DIRECTIONS

Brush Portobello caps with melted butter from all sides. Preheat the oven to 355F/180C. Line the tray with baking paper. Put Portobello caps on the tray. Beat the quail eggs into the mushroom caps and sprinkle them with salt and dried parsley. Transfer the tray to the oven. Cook the mushrooms for 15 minutes. Chill a little and transfer to the serving plates.

Nutrition:
- Calories: 191
- Fat: 4.4 g
- Fiber: 1.4 g
- Carbs: 5.3 g
- Protein: 17 g
- Cholesterol: 377 mg
- Sodium: 1036 mg

# Salmon Omelete

Servings: 2          Prep time: 10 min          Cook time: 8 min

INGREDIENTS

3 eggs
2 slices of smoked salmon
3 links of pork sausage
¼ cup of onions
¼ cup of provolone cheese

DIRECTIONS

Whisk the eggs and pour them into a skillet. Follow the standard method for making an omelet. Add the onions, salmon, and cheese before turning the omelet over. Sprinkle the omelet with cheese and serve with the sausages on the side.

Nutrition:
- Calories: 274
- Fat: 18.3 g
- Carbs: 2.2 g
- Protein: 24.2 g
- Cholesterol: 283 mg
- Sodium: 1234 mg

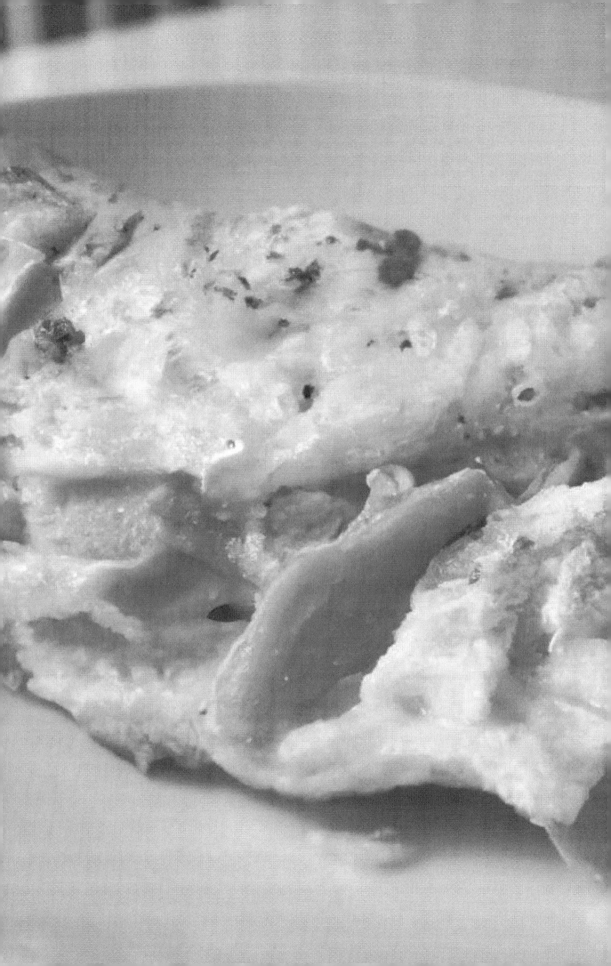

# Peanut Butter Bread

Servings: 2          Prep time: 15min          Cook time: 5 min

INGREDIENTS

1 tbsp of oil
2 tbsps of peanut butter
4 slices of bread
1 banana, sliced

DIRECTIONS

Spread the peanut butter on top of each slice of bread, then arrange the banana slices on top. Sandwich 2 pieces together, then the other two. Oil the inside of the Air Fryer and cook the bread for 5 minutes at 300F/149C.

Nutrition:
- Calories: 255
- Fat: 15.6 g
- Fiber: 2.9 g
- Carbs: 25.7 g
- Protein: 6 g
- Cholesterol: 0 mg
- Sodium: 197 mg

# Bacon Cups

Servings: 2          Prep time: 40 min          Cook time:20min

INGREDIENTS

2 eggs
1 tomato
3 slices of bacon
2 slices of ham
2 tsp of grated parmesan cheese

DIRECTIONS

Preheat your oven to 375F/190C. Fry the bacon in a pan till crisp. Slice the bacon strips in half and line 2 greased muffin tins with three half-strips of bacon. Put one slice of ham and half a tomato in each muffin tin on top of the bacon. Crack one egg on top of the tomato in each muffin tin and sprinkle each with half a tsp of grated parmesan cheese. Bake for 20 minutes. Remove and let cool.

Nutrition:
- Calories: 309
- Fat: 21.3 g
- Carbs: 2.6 g
- Protein: 25.2 g
- Cholesterol: 221 mg
- Sodium:1215 mg

# Toasties

Servings: 2          Prep time: 30min          Cook time: 20min

## INGREDIENTS

¼ cup of milk or cream

2 sausages, boiled

3 eggs

1 slice of bread, sliced lengthwise

4 tbsps of cheese, grated

Sea salt to taste

Chopped fresh herbs and steamed broccoli [optional]

Nutrition:
- Calories: 270
- Fat: 19.6 g
- Fiber: 0.2 g
- Carbs: 4.5 g
- Protein: 18.4 g
- Cholesterol: 286 mg
- Sodium: 427 mg

## DIRECTIONS

Preheat your Air Fryer to 360F/182F and set the timer for 5 minutes. In the meantime, scramble the eggs in a bowl and add the milk. Grease three muffin cups with cooking spray. Divide the egg mixture into three and pour equal amounts into each cup. Slice the sausages and drop them, along with the slices of bread, into the egg mixture. Add the cheese on top and a little salt as desired. Transfer the cups to the fryer and cook for 10-15 minutes, depending on how firm you want. You can also use an oven at 360F/182C for 20-30 minutes.

# Coffee Donuts

Servings: 2          Prep time: 20 min          Cook time:10min

## INGREDIENTS

1 cup of almond flour

¼ cup of stevia

salt

1 tsp of baking powder

1 tbsp of aquafaba=liquid leftover from cooked chickpeas

1 tbsp of olive oil

¼ cup of coffee

Nutrition:
- Calories: 405
- Fat: 33.3 g
- Carbs: 13.2 g
- Protein: 13 g
- Cholesterol: 0 mg
- Sodium: 32 mg

## DIRECTIONS

Combine the stevia, salt, flour, and baking powder in a large bowl. Mix the coffee, aquafaba, and oil until a dough is formed. Leave the dough to rest in the refrigerator. Set your Air Fryer at 400F/200C to heat up. Remove the dough from the fridge and divide it, kneading each section into a doughnut. Put the doughnuts inside the air fryer, ensuring not to overlap any. Fry for 6 minutes. Do not shake the basket to make sure the doughnuts hold their shape. You can fry them in deep oil if you do not have an air fryer.

# SALADS AND SOUPS

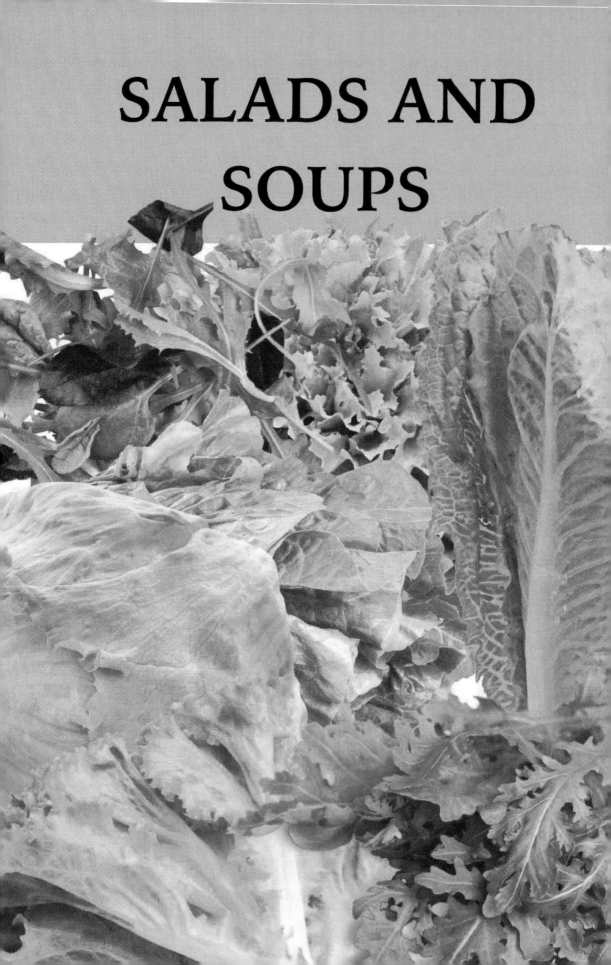

# Apple/Peach Salad

Servings: 2      Prep time: 4min      Cook time: 0min

## INGREDIENTS

2 chopped apples
1 cup of peach chopped
1 cup of blackberries
1 tbsp of lime juice
1 tbsp of honey
¼ tsp of dried thyme
salt

## DIRECTIONS

Toss all ingredients together and serve.

Nutrition:
- Calories: 211
- Fat: 1 g
- Fiber: 10.3 g
- Carbs: 54 g
- Protein: 2.3 g
- Cholesterol: 0 mg
- Sodium: 1165 mg

# Chicken/Apple Salad

Servings: 2      Prep time: 10 min      Cook time: 0min

## INGREDIENTS

2 cup of basil
1 cup of chopped apple
1 cup of cooked chopped chicken breast
½ cup of sliced red onion
¼ cup of chopped pecans
2 tbsp of Acai Dressing

## DIRECTIONS

Set 2 salad bowls on the table and add basil to each. Add each of your remaining ingredients as layers on top of the greens. Once ready, drizzle each bowl of salad with dressing.

Nutrition:
- Calories 679
- Fat: 52.5g
- Carbs: 31.2g
- Protein: 29.5g
- Cholesterol: 54mg
- Sodium: 48mg

# Avocado/Quinoa Salad

Servings: 2          Prep time: 10min          Cook time: 0min

INGREDIENTS

1½ cup of cooked quinoa
4 oz. of julienned cucumber
4 oz. of julienned carrots
½ diced avocado
½ cup of Brussels sprouts

DIRECTIONS

Split Quinoa into 2 medium bowls. Top with cucumber, avocado, and carrot. Add the blanched Brussel Sprouts. Mix and serve.

Nutrition:
- Calories: 640
- Fat: 16.2 g
- Fiber: 18.3 g
- Carbs: 106.8 g
- Protein: 21.3 g
- Cholesterol: 0 mg
- Sodium: 165 mg

# Kale Salad

Servings: 2          Prep time: 10 min          Cook time:0min

INGREDIENTS

1 bunch of chopped kale
1 cup of fresh peas
2 chopped carrots
1 cup of boiled potatoes
1 cup of sliced cabbage
2 tbsps of apple cider vinegar
1 tsp of chili powder
salt
2 tbsps of coconut oil
1 tsp of coconut powder

DIRECTIONS

Combine all vegetables in a bowl. Drizzle with vinegar and coconut oil. Season with salt and chili powder. Sprinkle with coconut powder and toss to combine. Add to a serving dish and serve.

Nutrition:
- Calories 287
- Fat: 14.8 g
- Carbs: 35.1 g
- Protein: 7.1 g
- Cholesterol: 0
- Sodium: 667 mg

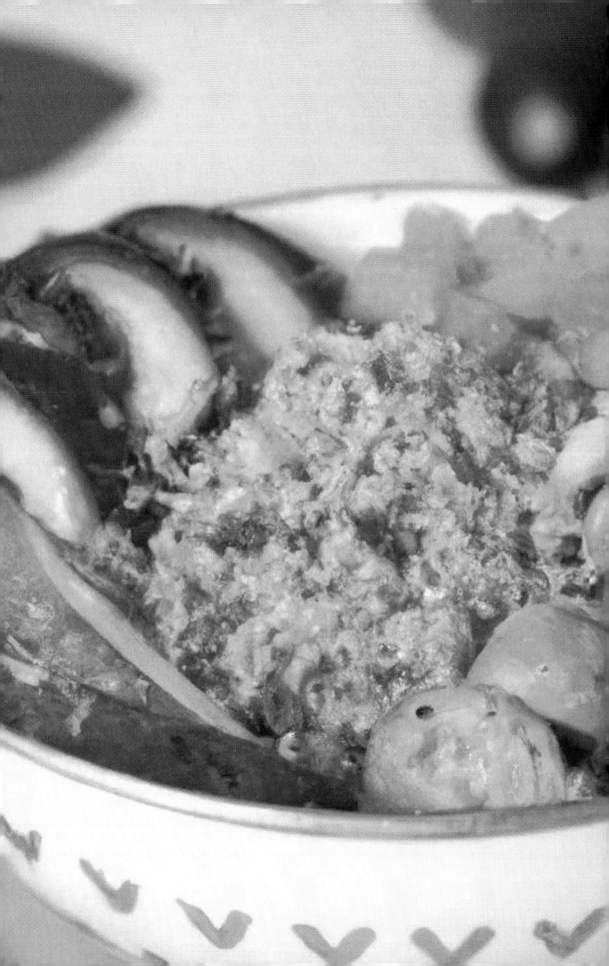

# Strawberry Lentil Salad

Servings: 2          Prep time: 35min          Cook time: 20min

INGREDIENTS

1/2 cup lentils
1/2 cup edamame
1 rhubarb sticks (young)
1/2 cup strawberries,
1/2 cup Snow peas,
1 tbsp sesame seed oil
1 tbsp lemon juice
bunch of basil
½ cup bocconcini (small fresh mozzarella balls)

Nutrition:
- Calories: 379
- Fat: 13.2 g
- Fiber: 19.7 g
- Carbs: 43.1 g
- Protein: 24.5 g
- Cholesterol: 4 mg
- Sodium: 60 mg

DIRECTIONS

Boil the lentils, drain them, and let them cool. Boil the edamame for 5 minutes in salted water. Drain and cool before removing the edamame from the pods. Prepare the rhubarb and strawberries by washing, cleaning, and slicing them. Snow peas should be washed, cleaned, and cut in half diagonally. Combine sesame oil, lemon juice, salt, and pepper in a large mixing bowl. Basil should be washed, dried, and coarsely chopped. Add all ingredients together with the dressing and divide among 2 bowls. Distribute the mozzarella among the bowls.

# Peas Salad

Servings: 2          Prep time: 20 min          Cook time:30min

INGREDIENTS

1 cups green peas
1/2 cup of sweetcorn drained
1 medium carrot peeled and grated
2 spring onions finely chopped
for the sauce:
2 tbsp olive oil
1/2 tbsp balsamic vinegar
1 tiny chili seeds removed, finely chopped
1/2 tsp minced garlic
juice of 1 lime
a handful of parsley roughly chopped

DIRECTIONS

Use dried peas, and boil them for about 30 minutes. Drain and leave to cool. If you use canned peas: empty the contents into a colander. Rinse with cold water and drain well. Combine all ingredients for the dressing in a large bowl and season with black pepper to taste. Mix well with the sauce over the peas, sweet corn, and grated carrot. Add chopped spring onions to garnish.

Nutrition:
- Calories: 286
- Fat: 15.7 g
- Carbs: 34 g
- Protein: 8 g
- Cholesterol: 0 mg
- Sodium: 28 mg

46

# Rice Salad

Servings: 2          Prep time: 35min          Cook time: 20min

## INGREDIENTS

1 cup of rice,
1/2 cup of pickles,
1/2 cup of tuna in oil,
1/2 cup of cheese
2 eggs,
2 tbsps of olives,
1 tbsp mayonnaise,
extra virgin olive oil

Nutrition:
- Calories: 580
- Fat: 35 g
- Fiber: 1.7 g
- Carbs: 33.1 g
- Protein: 32 g
- Cholesterol: 234 mg
- Sodium: 1145 mg

## DIRECTIONS

Cut the pickles into tiny pieces. Cut a cheese of your choice into small cubes. Boil the eggs for 10 minutes. Boil the rice in hot, salted water for the time indicated on the package. Once cooked, drain it, pass it under a large jet of cold water to cool it, transfer it to a big salad bowl, and immediately add a little oil to prevent it from sticking. Add the drained and chopped tuna, the pickles, and the pitted olives, mix, and place in a container. Let it cool for an hour. Add the chopped cheese, boiled eggs, and mayonnaise with olive oil when the rice is cold, and mix everything well.

# Banana Salad

Servings: 2          Prep time: 5 min          Cook time: 0min

## INGREDIENTS

4 sliced bananas
¼ cup of pineapple sauce
1 tbsp of lime juice
¼ tsp of cinnamon powder
¼ tsp of chili flakes

## DIRECTIONS

Add bananas, pineapple sauce, lemon juice, and mix in a bowl. Season with cinnamon and chili flakes.

Nutrition:
- Calories: 210
- Fat: 0.8 g
- Carbs: 53 g
- Protein: 2.6 g
- Cholesterol: 0 mg
- Sodium: 2 mg

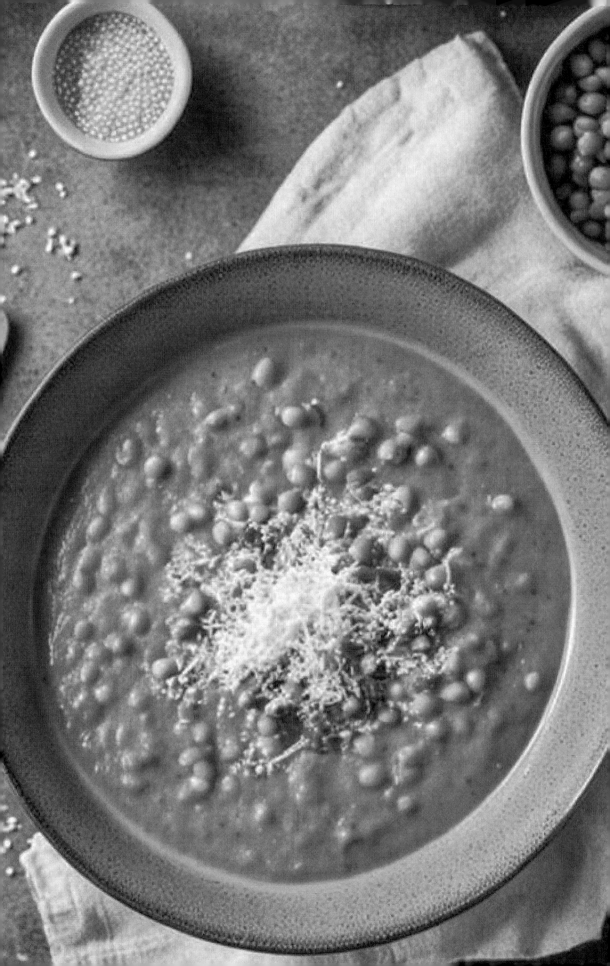

# Pea Soup

Servings: 2          Prep time: 20min          Cook time: 15min

## INGREDIENTS

1 shallot
1 garlic clove
2 tbsp olive oil
1 cup peas (frozen)
1 cup vegetable broth
4 dill stems
½ cup feta cheese
½ cup whipped light cream
Chili flakes (optional)
1 tbsp sesame seeds

Nutrition:
- Calories: 416
- Fat: 34.6 g
- Fiber: 4.3 g
- Carbs: 15.8 g
- Protein: 13.4 g
- Cholesterol: 67 mg
- Sodium: 815 mg

## DIRECTIONS

Peel the garlic and shallot. Heat 1 tbsp of oil, sauté shallots, and garlic for 3 minutes over medium heat in a saucepan. Cook for another 3 minutes. After adding the peas, add the vegetable stock and cook for 5 minutes. Meanwhile, wash and dry the dill before plucking it into small bits. Using your hands, crumble the feta cheese. Next, pour the cream and finely puree the soup with half of the dill using a hand blender: salt, pepper, and chili flakes to taste in the pea soup. Fill two bowls with the remaining dill, feta, and sesame seeds, and drizzle with the remaining oil.

# Lentil and Potato Soup

Servings: 2          Prep time: 20 min          Cook time:20min

## INGREDIENTS

2 carrots
1/2 cup potatoes
2 tbsp olive oil
½ cup red lentil
2 tbsp turmeric powder
2 cups vegetable broth
1 tbsp Tomato paste
cayenne
1 tbsp whipped cream
2 slices wholemeal sourdough bread
1 handful basil fresh

Nutrition:
- Calories 524
- Fat: 19.5 g
- Carbs: 65.9 g
- Protein: 23.2 g
- Cholesterol: 8 0mg
- Sodium: 1031 mg

## DIRECTIONS

Peel and cut the carrots and potatoes into small cubes. Heat 1 tbsp of oil in a saucepan, add carrots and potatoes and saute for 4 minutes over medium heat. Cook for 2 minutes after adding the lentils and turmeric. Season with salt and pepper, and add vegetable stock and tomato paste. Boil for 15 minutes over low heat. Using a hand blender, puree in cream. Dice bread slices simultaneously. In a separate pan, heat the remaining oil. Over medium heat, toast the bread cubes for 5 minutes or until golden brown. Clean the basil leaves by shaking them dry and plucking their leaves. Fill bowls halfway with broth, drizzle with cream, and top with bread cubes and basil.

# Veggie Soup

INGREDIENTS

1 tbsp of olive oil
1 chopped yellow onion
2 chopped celery ribs
2 chopped carrots
2 zucchini, chopped
1 cup cauliflower florets
black pepper
1 tsp of dried thyme
½ tsp of garlic powder
1 tsp of dried oregano
4 cub of veggie stock
1 bay leaf
14 oz. of chopped canned tomatoes

DIRECTIONS

Add the oil to a pot and heat over medium-high heat; add onion, celery, and carrots, stir, and sauté them for 4 minutes. Add all other vegetables, spices, and stock, stir, simmer, and cook for 20 minutes. Stir the soup again, ladle it into bowls, and serve.

Nutrition:
- Calories: 182
- Fat: 6.2 g
- Fiber: 8.3 g
- Carbs: 23.8 g
- Protein: 3.3 g
- Cholesterol: 0 mg
- Sodium: 499 mg

# Pumpkin Soup

INGREDIENTS

1 chopped yellow onion
¾ cup of water
2 cups  pumpkin puree
2 cups of veggie stock
½ tsp of cinnamon powder
¼ tsp of ground nutmeg
1 cup of fat-free milk
Black pepper
1 chopped green onion

DIRECTIONS

Put the water in a pot, simmer over medium heat, add onion, stock, and pumpkin puree, and stir. Add the cinnamon, nutmeg, milk, and black pepper. Stir, cook for 10 minutes, ladle into bowls, sprinkle green onion on top, and serve.

Nutrition:
- Calories 153
- Fat: 2.8 g
- Carbs: 31.1 g
- Protein: 7.1 g
- Cholesterol: 2 mg
- Sodium: 802 mg

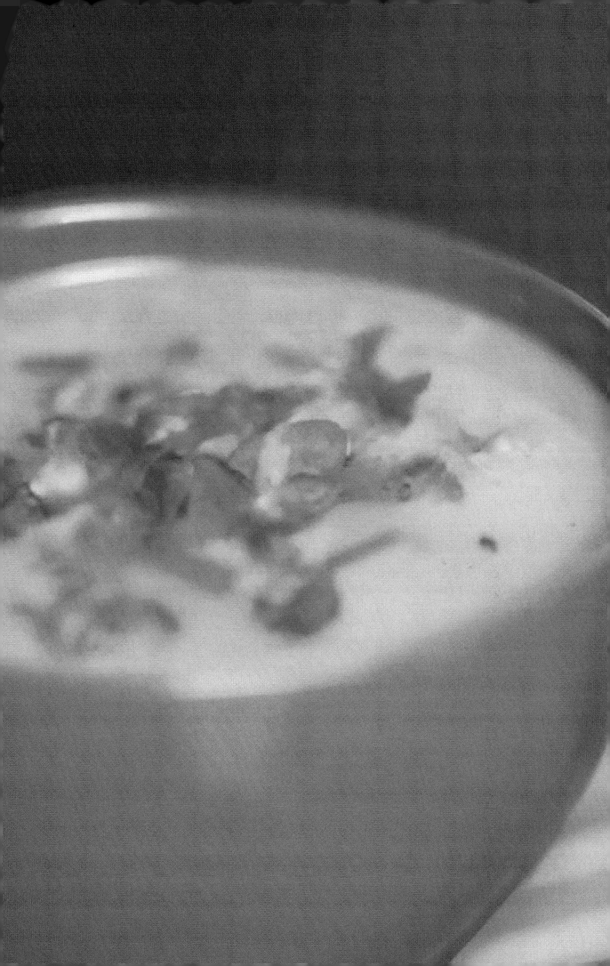

# Shrimp Soup

Servings: 2     Prep time: 10min     Cook time: 25min

## INGREDIENTS

8 oz. of shrimp
1 stalk lemongrass
2 grated ginger
6 cup of low-sodium chicken stock
2 chopped jalapenos
4 lime leaves
1½ cup of chopped pineapple
1 cup of chopped shiitake mushroom caps
1 chopped tomato
½ cubed bell pepper
1 tsp of stevia
¼ cup of lime juice
1/3 cup of chopped cilantro
2 sliced scallions
1 tbsp fish sauce

## DIRECTIONS

Mix ginger with lemongrass, stock, jalapenos, and lime leaves in a pot. Stir, boil over medium heat, cover, cook for 15 minutes, strain liquid in a bowl, and discard solids. Return the soup to the pot, and add pineapple, tomato, mushrooms, bell pepper, sugar, and fish sauce. Stir, boil over medium heat, cook for 5 minutes, add shrimp, and cook for 3 more minutes. Add the lime juice, cilantro, and scallions, stir, ladle into soup bowls, and serve.

Nutrition:
- Calories: 491
- Fat: 3.5 g
- Fiber: 11.3 g
- Carbs: 88.8 g
- Protein: 35.3 g
- Cholesterol: 239 mg
- Sodium: 1395 mg

# Chestnut Soup

Servings: 2     Prep time: 10 min     Cook time:40min

## INGREDIENTS

2 cups of whole roasted chestnuts
1 chopped shallot
½ cup of light cream
½ cup of chicken stock
1 chopped leek
¼ cup of chopped carrots
2 tbsp of olive oil
1 sprig thyme
1 bay leaf
1 chopped celery stalk
½ tsp of nutmeg
Salt, Pepper

Nutrition:
- Calories 271
- Fat: 23.2 g
- Carbs: 15.1 g
- Protein: 2.1 g
- Cholesterol: 72 mg
- Sodium: 310 mg

## DIRECTIONS

Add the oil, carrot, leek, shallot, and celery in a saucepan over medium heat. Cook for 6-7 minutes or until the vegetables are tender. Add the stock, thyme, bay leaf, and chestnuts, and boil. Reduce heat and simmer for 25 minutes. Remove from the heat and discard the thyme and bay leaf. Allow to cool slightly, and puree using an immersion blender. Heat the soup as you stir the cream and nutmeg, and season to taste. Cook for 5 minutes more. Serve hot.

# Tuna/Squished Salad

Servings: 2          Prep time: 10min          Cook time: 10min

## INGREDIENTS

2 tsp Cajun seasoning
2 tuna steaks
1cup cherry tomatoes halved
1cup baby leaf spinach
1cup mangetout halved lengthways

Nutrition:
- Calories: 249
- Fat: 2.4 g
- Fiber: 2.9 g
- Carbs: 10.3 g
- Protein: 46,6 g
- Cholesterol: 75 mg
- Sodium: 115 mg

## DIRECTIONS

Sprinkle the Cajun seasoning over the tuna steaks and fry for 2 minutes on each side in a nonstick pan over high heat. If you prefer your tuna cooked all through, get it for 3 minutes on each side. Squish the tomatoes slightly in a large bowl using a fork so that you catch all the juices. Stir in the spinach and mangetout and season to taste. Pile the salad onto plates and top with the tuna steaks to serve.

# Tuna Salad

Servings: 2          Prep time: 5min          Cook time:0min

## INGREDIENTS

5 oz. of tuna
1 tbsp of extra virgin olive oil
1 tbsp of red wine vinegar
$\frac{1}{4}$ cup of chopped green onion
2 cups of arugula
1 cup of cooked pasta
1 tbsp of Parmesan cheese
Black pepper

Nutrition:
- Calories 582
- Fat: 16.2 g
- Carbs: 71.9 g
- Protein: 35 g
- Cholesterol: 117 mg
- Sodium: 118 mg

## DIRECTIONS

Combine all your ingredients in a medium bowl and mix well. Split the mixture between two plates.

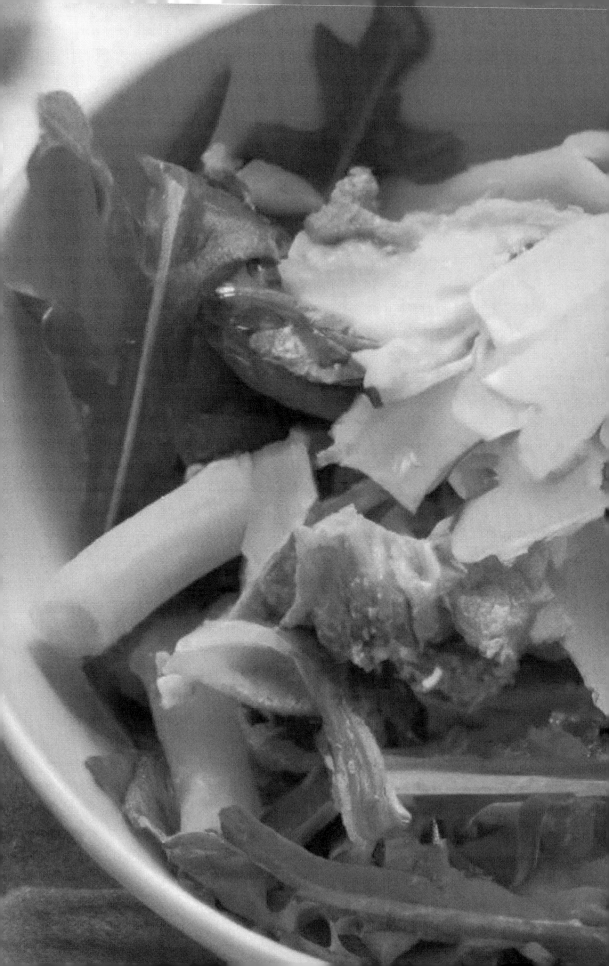

# SEAFOOD

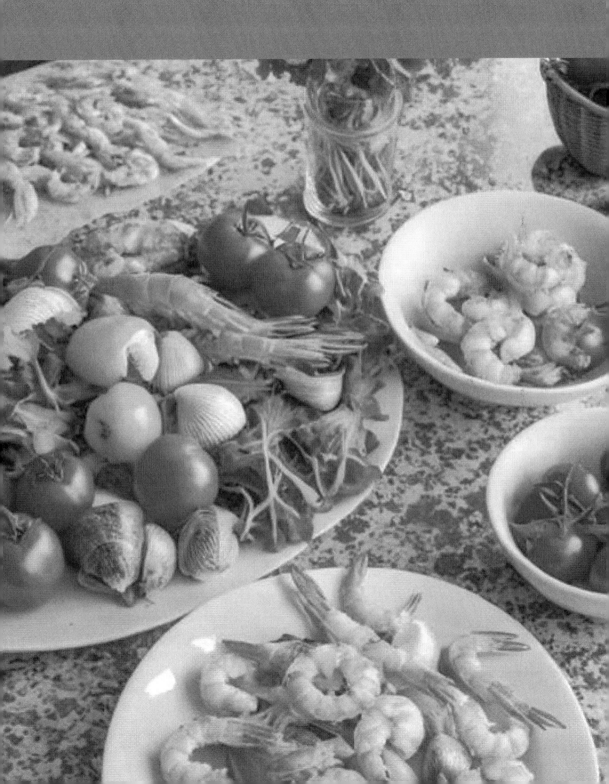

# Steamed Salmon

Servings: 2　　　Prep time: 10min　　　Cook time: 15min

## INGREDIENTS

3 green onions, minced
2 packet of Stevia
1 tbsp of freshly grated ginger
1 clove of garlic, minced
2 tsp of sesame seeds
1 tbsp of sesame oil
¼ cup of mirin
2 tbsps of low sodium soy sauce
1/2-lb. of salmon filet

Nutrition:
- Calories: 606
- Fat: 31 g
- Fiber: 1.5 g
- Carbs: 23.3 g
- Protein: 56.3 g
- Cholesterol: 158 mg
- Sodium: 993 mg

## DIRECTIONS

Place a large saucepan on medium-high heat. Place a trivet inside the saucepan and fill the pan halfway with water. Cover and bring to a boil. Meanwhile, mix stevia, ginger, garlic, oil, mirin, and soy sauce in a heatproof dish that fits inside the saucepan. Add salmon and cover generously with the sauce. Top the salmon with sesame seeds and green onions. Cover the dish with foil. Place on top of the trivet and steam for 15 minutes. Let it rest for 5 minutes in the pan before serving.

# Dill and Cod

Servings: 2　　　Prep time: 10min　　　Cook time: 10min

## INGREDIENTS

2 tsp of olive oil, divided
4 slices of lemon, divided
2 sprigs of fresh dill, divided
½ tsp of garlic powder, divided
Pepper to taste
1/2-lb. of cod filets

Nutrition:
- Calories: 401
- Fat: 25.2 g
- Carbs: 133,6 g
- Protein: 17.7 g
- Cholesterol: 34 mg
- Sodium: 2500 mg

## DIRECTIONS

Place a large saucepan on the medium-high fire. Place a trivet inside the saucepan and fill the pan halfway with water. Cover and bring to a boil. Cut 2 pieces of 15-inch length foil. Place one filet in the middle. Season with pepper to taste in one foil. Sprinkle ¼ tsp of garlic. Add a tsp of oil on top of the filet. Top with 2 slices of lemon and a sprig of dill. Fold over the foil and seal the filet inside. Repeat the process for the remaining fish. Cover the packets on the trivet and steam for 10 minutes.

# Salmon with Beetroot

Servings: 2        Prep time: 20min        Cook time: 60min

## INGREDIENTS

1 cup beetroot peeled and diced
2 boneless salmon fillets
2 cups potatoes halved or quartered
2 tbsp fromage frais
2 level tsp horseradish sauce

Nutrition:
- Calories: 541
- Fat: 20 g
- Fiber: 6.5 g
- Carbs: 44,9 g
- Protein: 45 g
- Cholesterol: 108 mg
- Sodium: 243 mg

## DIRECTIONS

Preheat the oven to 400F/200C and line a tray with baking paper. Boil the beetroot in a large covered saucepan, for 25 minutes or until tender. Add the potatoes to the beetroot pan for the last 15 minutes of the cooking time, topping up the water if necessary. Arrange the salmon fillets on the baking tray and season lightly. Bake for 15 minutes or until cooked. Mix the fromage frais and horseradish in a large bowl and season lightly. Drain the potatoes and beetroot, rinse under cold running water, and drain again. Tip into the bowl of dressing, then toss well and put on plates with the salmon. Grind over some black pepper to serve.

# Crab Lettuce Cups

Servings: 2        Prep time: 10min        Cook time:25min

## INGREDIENTS

1 cup dried basmati and wild rice
1 can white crabmeat drained
2 tbsp fromage frais
½ small pack fresh coriander roughly chopped
3 little gem lettuces leaves separated

Nutrition:
- Calories: 343
- Fat: 8.6 g
- Carbs: 3,6 g
- Protein: 30.7 g
- Cholesterol: 83 mg
- Sodium: 535 mg

## DIRECTIONS

Rinse the rice under cold running water, tip it into a saucepan, and cover it with cold water. Season with salt, boil over high heat and simmer for 20-25 minutes or until tender. Drain and leave to cool. Mix the crab, fromage frais, and coriander and season to taste. Finely shred any lettuce leaves that are too small to stuff and stir them into the crab mixture. Stir the cooled rice into the crab mixture and spoon the mixture into the lettuce leaves to serve.

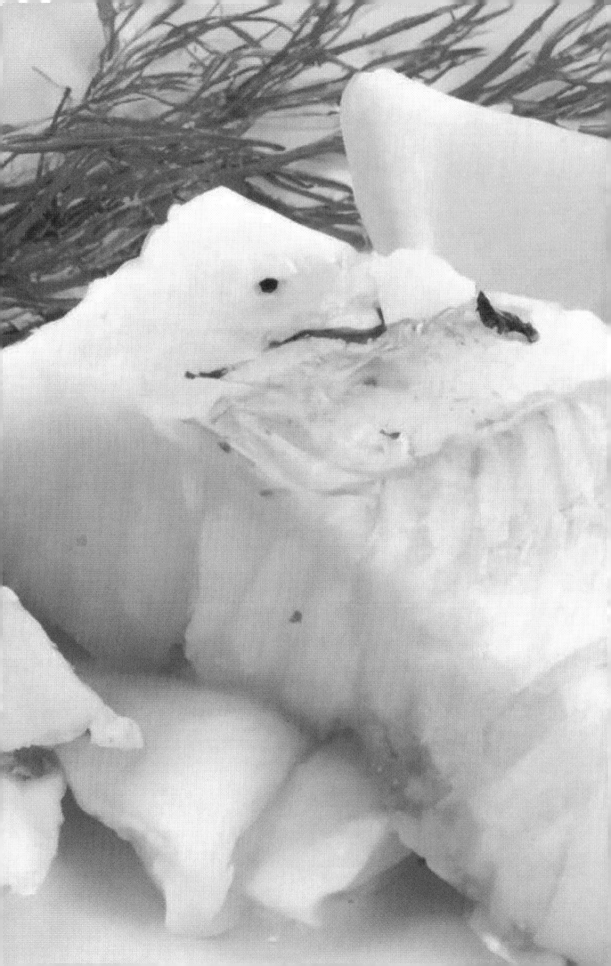

# Seafood Pancake

Servings: 2          Prep time: 10min          Cook time: 10min

## INGREDIENTS

4 spring onions thinly sliced
1 cup seafood selection
thawed if frozen
1 garlic clove crushed
1 cup mixed stir fry
vegetables
4 eggs

Nutrition:
- Calories: 270
- Fat: 15.9 g
- Fiber: 1.5 g
- Carbs: 1.7 g
- Protein: 50.3 g
- Cholesterol: 460 mg
- Sodium: 160 mg

## DIRECTIONS

Place a nonstick frying pan over medium heat. Add the spring onions, seafood, garlic, and vegetables and stir fry for 3-4 minutes or until piping hot. Preheat the grill to hot. Lightly beat the eggs, season, and pour over the fish mixture. Fry for 2-3 minutes or until the bottom is set, then finish under the grill for 1-2 minutes or until crispy and golden. Serve hot.

# Spaghetti with Salmon

Servings: 2          Prep time: 10min          Cook time:25min

## INGREDIENTS

1 cup spaghetti
grated zest and juice of 1
large lemon
1cup smoked salmon, sliced
1 large red chilli deseeded
and shopped
small bag of rocket leaves

Nutrition:
- Calories: 477
- Fat: 7.2 g
- Carbs: 68.4 g
- Protein: 32.4 g
- Cholesterol: 114 mg
- Sodium: 2033 mg

## DIRECTIONS

Cook the pasta according to the pack instructions. Mix the lemon juice, salmon chilli, and rocket in a bowl. Drain the pasta and return to the saucepan; toss the salmon mixture, divide between shallow bowls, and scatter with lemon zest to serve.

# Steamed Cod

Servings: 2      Prep time: 10min      Cook time: 20min

## INGREDIENTS

Pepper to taste
1 clove of garlic, smashed
2 tsp of olive oil
1 bunch of fresh thyme
2 tbsps of pickled capers
1 cup of black salt-cured olives
1 cup of cherry tomatoes halved
2 pcs cod filets

Nutrition:
- Calories: 150
- Fat: 5,2 g
- Fiber: 1.5 g
- Carbs: 0.5 g
- Protein: 50.3 g
- Cholesterol: 0 mg
- Sodium: 79,5 mg

## DIRECTIONS

Place a large saucepan on the medium-high. Place a trivet inside the saucepan and fill the pan halfway with water. Cover and bring to a boil. Meanwhile, layer half of the halved cherry tomatoes in a heatproof dish that fits inside the saucepan—season with pepper. Add the filets to the tomatoes, season with pepper, and drizzle oil. Sprinkle 3/4 of thyme on top and the smashed garlic. Cover the top of the fish with the remaining cherry tomatoes plus the capers and olives, then place the dish on the trivet. Cover the dish with foil. Cover the pan and steam for 15 minutes.

# Steamed Tilapia

Servings: 2      Prep time: 10min      Cook time:15min

## INGREDIENTS

2 pcs Tilapia filets
1 tsp of garlic
1 tsp of minced ginger
2 tbsp of rice wine
1 tbsp of low sodium soy sauce

Nutrition:
- Calories: 328
- Fat: 6.7 g
- Carbs: 8,9 g
- Protein: 59.3 g
- Cholesterol: 133 mg
- Sodium: 13110 mg

## DIRECTIONS

Add garlic, minced ginger, rice wine, and soy sauce in a heatproof dish that fits inside the saucepan. Mix well. Add the Tilapia filet and marinate for half an hour while turning it over at half-time. Place a large saucepan on the medium-high fire. Place a trivet inside the saucepan and fill the pan halfway with water. Cover and bring to a boil. Cover the dish of fish with foil and place it on a trivet. Cover the pan and steam for 15 minutes.

60

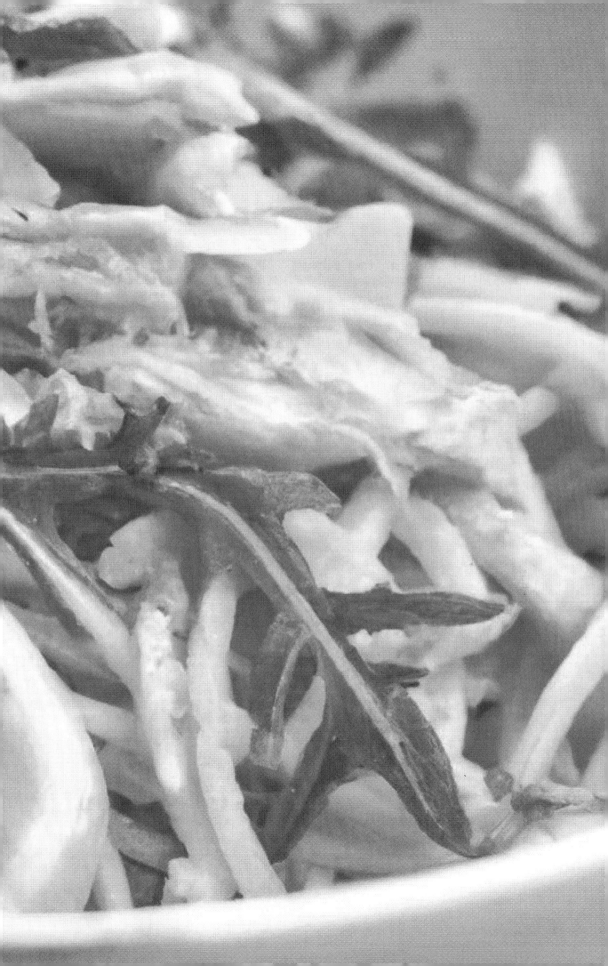

# Stewed Cod Fish

Servings: 2　　　Prep time: 10min　　　Cook time: 15min

## INGREDIENTS

1 tbsp of olive oil

1 onion, sliced

2 fresh cod fillets

Pepper

1 lemon juice, freshly squeezed

1 can of diced tomatoes

## DIRECTIONS

Place a heavy-bottomed pot on medium-high fire and heat for 3 minutes. Once hot, add oil and stir around to coat the pot with oil. Sauté the onion for 2 minutes. Stir in diced tomatoes and cook for 5 minutes. Add the cod filet and season with pepper. Cover, boil, lower the fire, and simmer for 5 minutes. Serve with freshly squeezed lemon juice.

Nutrition:
- Calories: 198
- Fat: 7.7 g
- Fiber: 0 g
- Carbs: 8.7 g
- Protein: 1.4 g
- Cholesterol: 0 mg
- Sodium: 86 mg

# Tuna Casserole

Servings: 2　　　Prep time: 10min　　　Cook time: 12min

## INGREDIENTS

2 carrots, peeled and chopped

$\frac{1}{4}$ cup of diced onions

1 cup of frozen peas

$\frac{3}{4}$ cup of milk

2 cans of tuna in water, drained

1 can of cream of celery soup

1 tbsp of olive oil

$\frac{1}{2}$ cup of water

2 eggs beaten

Pepper

## DIRECTIONS

Place a heavy-bottomed pot on medium-high heat for 3 minutes. Once hot, add the oil and stir around to coat the pot with oil. Sauté the onion and carrots for 3 minutes. Add the remaining ingredients and mix well. Bring to a boil while constantly stirring. Cook until thickened, around 5 minutes.

Nutrition:
- Calories: 600
- Fat: 26.2 g
- Carbs: 34.6 g
- Protein: 56.7 g
- Cholesterol: 283 mg
- Sodium: 1456 mg

# Seafood Recipe

Servings: 2     Prep time: 10min     Cook time: 20min

## INGREDIENTS

3 onions, chopped
2 cloves of garlic, minced
1-inch of ginger, grated
1 tsp of oil
3 cups of water
1 2-inch of long kombu or dried kelp
6 shiitake mushrooms, halved
12 manila clams, scrubbed
1 cup of medium-sized shrimps, peeled and deveined
1 cup of bay scallops
1 package of Japanese curry roux
1/4 apple, sliced

## DIRECTIONS

Place a heavy-bottomed pot on medium-high heat for 3 minutes. Once hot, add oil and stir around to coat the pot with oil. Sauté the onion, ginger, and garlic for 5 minutes. Add the remaining ingredients and mix well. Cover, boil, lower the fire, and simmer for 5 minutes. Let it rest for 5 minutes.

Nutrition:
- Calories: 607
- Fat: 1.7 g
- Fiber: 9 g
- Carbs: 57.3 g
- Protein: 78 g
- Cholestero: 565 mg
- Sodium: 1296 mg

# Shrimps and Asparagus

Servings: 2     Prep time: 10min   Cook time:15min

## INGREDIENTS

1cup of shrimp, peeled and deveined
1 bunch of asparagus, trimmed
1 tsp of oil
1/2 tbsp of Cajun seasoning

## DIRECTIONS

Add all the ingredients to a heatproof dish that fits inside the saucepan. Mix well. Place a large saucepan on medium-high fire. Place a trivet inside the saucepan and fill the pan halfway with water. Cover and bring to a boil. Cover the dish with foil and place on the trivet. Cover the pan and steam for 10 minutes. Let it rest in the pan for another 5 minutes.

Nutrition:
- Calories: 303
- Fat: 6.2 g
- Carbs: 6 g
- Protein: 53,2 g
- Cholesterol: 478 mg
- Sodium: 592 mg

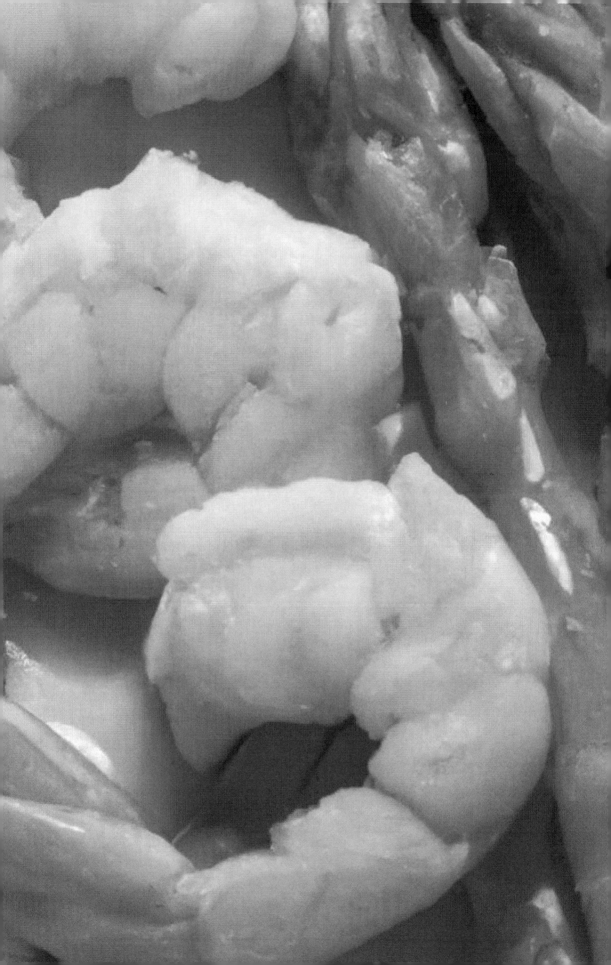

# Baked Cod

Servings: 2          Prep time: 40min          Cook time: 30min

INGREDIENTS

2 cod fillets

1 cup of Brussels sprouts

1 tbsp of olive oil

Salt and black pepper to taste

1 cup of crème Fraiche

2 tbsps of Parmesan cheese, grated

2 tbsps of shaved almonds

Nutrition:
- Calories: 881
- Fat: 74.9 g
- Fiber: 3.5 g
- Carbs: 13.3 g
- Protein: 38.5 g
- Cholesterol: 215 mg
- Sodium: 482 mg

DIRECTIONS

Toss the fish fillets and Brussels sprouts in oil and season with salt and black pepper to taste. Spread in a greased baking dish. Mix the crème Fraiche with Parmesan cheese, and pour and smear the cream on the fish. Bake in the oven for 25 minutes at 400F/200C until golden brown. Take the dish out, sprinkle with the almonds, and bake for another 5 minutes. Best served hot.

# Salmon with Broccoli

Servings: 2          Prep time:30min          Cook time:25min

INGREDIENTS

2 salmon fillets

Salt and black pepper to taste

2 tbsps of mayonnaise

2 tbsps of fennel seeds, crushed

½ head of broccoli, cut in florets

1 red bell pepper, sliced

¼ cup chopped carrots

1 tbsp of olive oil

2 lemon wedges

Nutrition:
- Calories: 415
- Fat: 24.2 g
- Carbs: 16.1 g
- Protein: 37.7 g
- Cholesterol: 82 mg
- Sodium: 214 mg

DIRECTIONS

Brush the salmon with mayonnaise and season with salt and black pepper. Coat with fennel seeds, place in a lined baking dish and bake for 15 minutes at 370F/190C. Steam the broccoli and carrot for 3-4 minutes, or until tender, in a pot over medium flame. Heat the olive oil in a saucepan and sauté the red bell pepper for 5 minutes. Stir in the broccoli and turn off the heat. Let the pan sit for 2-3 minutes. Serve with baked salmon garnished with lemon wedges.

# Tuna Omelet Wraps

Servings: 2          Prep time: 15min          Cook time:15min

## INGREDIENTS

1 avocado, sliced
1 tbsp of chopped chives
1/3 cup of canned tuna, drained
2 spring onions, sliced
4 eggs, beaten in bowl
4 tbsps of mascarpone cheese
1 tbsp of butter
Salt and black pepper

Nutrition:
- Calories: 496
- Fat: 40.6 g
- Fiber: 7.2 g
- Carbs: 11.5 g
- Protein: 24.7 g
- Cholesterol: 368 mg
- Sodium: 213 mg

## DIRECTIONS

Combine the chives and mascarpone cheese; set aside. Melt the butter in a pan over medium heat. Add the eggs to the pan and cook for about 3 minutes. Flip the omelet over and continue cooking for another 2 minutes until golden. Season with salt and black pepper. Remove the omelet to a plate and spread the chive mixture over. Arrange the tuna, avocado, and onion slices. Wrap the omelet and serve immediately.

# Trout with Asparagus

Servings: 2          Prep time:30min          Cook time:15min

## INGREDIENTS

1 cup of asparagus spears
1 tbsp of garlic puree
2 pcs of deboned trout, butterflied
Salt and black pepper to taste
3 tbsps of olive oil
2 sprigs of rosemary
2 sprigs of thyme
2 tbsps of olive oil
½ medium red onion, sliced
2 lemon slices

## DIRECTIONS

Preheat the oven to 400F/200C. Rub the trout with garlic puree, salt, and black pepper. Prepare two aluminum foil squares. Place the fish on each square. Divide the asparagus and onion between the squares, and top with a pinch of salt and pepper, a sprig of rosemary and thyme, and 1 tbsp of oil. Also, lay the lemon slices on the fish. Wrap and close the fish packets securely, and place them on a baking sheet. Bake in the oven for 15 minutes.

Nutrition:
- Calories: 532
- Fat: 42 g
- Carbs: 9.1 g
- Protein: 35.2 g
- Cholesterol: 121mg
- Sodium: 166 mg

66

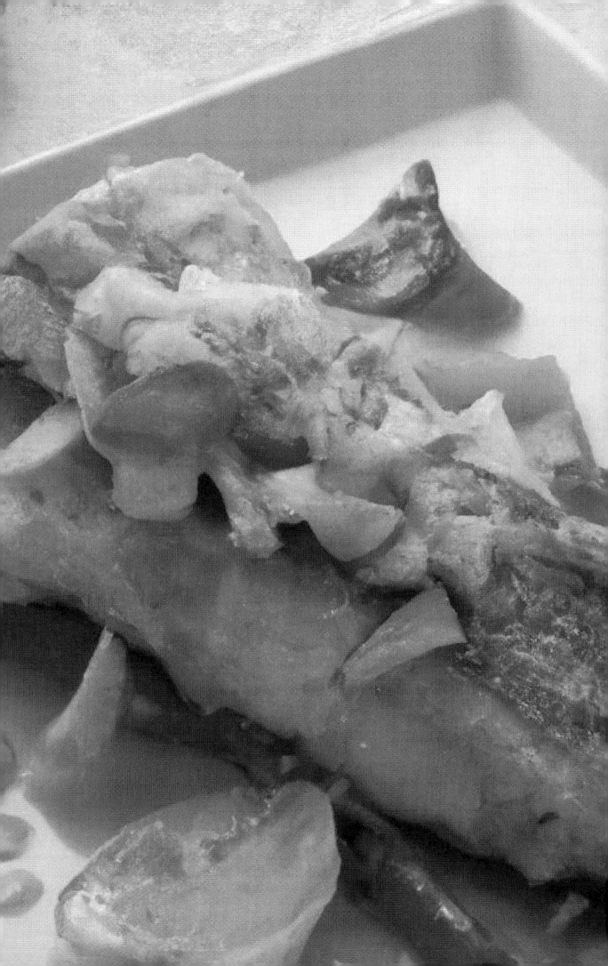

# Sea Bass

Servings: 2          Prep time: 25min          Cook time: 25min

INGREDIENTS

1 tbsp of olive oil

1 cup of red onions, sliced

2 bell peppers, deveined and sliced

Sea salt and cayenne pepper, to taste

1 tsp of paprika

2 pcs of sea bass fillets

Dill Sauce:

1 tbsp of mayonnaise

1/4 cup of Greek yogurt

1 tbsp of fresh dill, chopped

1/2 tsp of garlic powder

1/2 fresh lemon, juiced

DIRECTIONS

Toss the onions, peppers, and sea bass fillets with olive oil, salt, cayenne pepper, and paprika. Line a baking pan with a piece of parchment paper. Preheat your oven to 400F/200C. Arrange your fish and vegetables on the prepared baking pan. Bake for 10 minutes; turn them over and bake for 10 to 12 minutes. Meanwhile, make the sauce by mixing all ingredients until well combined. Serve the fish and vegetables with the dill sauce on the side.

Nutrition:
- Calories: 463
- Fat: 16.4 g
- Fiber: 3.9 g
- Carbs: 20.5 g
- Protein: 58.8 g
- Cholesterol: 123 mg
- Sodium: 267 mg

# Shrimp Stir

Servings: 2          Prep time:10min          Cook time:20min

INGREDIENTS

¼ cup of avocado oil

¼ cup of coconut aminos

2 cups of chopped broccoli

1 onion, diced

1 red bell pepper, chopped

1cup cooked and peeled shrimps

2 cups of cauliflower

Chili sauce, for serving (optional)

DIRECTIONS

Combine the shrimp, cauliflower, onion, pepper, broccoli, coconut aminos, and avocado oil in a large skillet. Cook, occasionally stirring, until all the flavors are combined, about 20 minutes. Drizzle the chili sauce over the top and serve hot.

Nutrition:
- Calories: 555
- Fat: 16.9 g
- Carbs: 52.9 g
- Protein: 57.9 g
- Cholesterol: 453 mg
- Sodium: 716 mg

# Salmon with Walnuts

Servings: 2          Prep time: 10min          Cook time: 12min

## INGREDIENTS

2 pcs of skinless salmon fillet

1/2 tsp of minced garlic

1 tsp of chopped fresh rosemary

salt

¼ tsp of crushed red pepper

½ tsp of honey

¼ tsp of lemon zest

1 tsp of lemon juice

1 tsp of olive oil and more as needed

2 tsps of Dijon mustard

3 tbsps of panko breadcrumbs

3 tbsps of finely chopped walnuts

## DIRECTIONS

Preheat oven to 425F/220C. Line a rimmed baking sheet with parchment paper, and place the skinless salmon fillet. Combine the minced garlic, chopped rosemary, salt, crushed red pepper, honey, lemon zest and juice, olive oil, mustard, and finely chopped walnuts. Rub the mixture on the fillet and then sprinkle with panko breadcrumbs. Grease the fish with olive oil baking spray and place the baking sheet into the oven. Bake for 8 to 12 minutes or until the fish is golden brown and cooked. Serve warm.

Nutrition:
- Calories: 424
- Fat: 37 g
- Fiber: 1.6 g
- Carbs: 5.6 g
- Protein: 36.5 g
- Cholesterol: 97 mg
- Sodium: 754 mg

# Salmon with Fennel

Servings: 2          Prep time:10min          Cook time:25min

## INGREDIENTS

2 pcs of salmon fillets,

1/4 tsp of ground pepper

4 tbsps of dry tomato pesto divided

2 medium fennel bulbs cut into 1/2-inch wedges

1 cup of couscous

3 scallions, thinly sliced

1/4 cup of sliced green olives

1 tsp of minced garlic

1 tbsp of olive oil, divided

1 lemon

1 tbsp of toasted pine nuts

½ cup of chicken broth

salt

Nutrition:
- Calories: 1764
- Fat: 62.6 g
- Carbs: 164,8 g
- Protein: 144.2 g
- Cholesterol: 275 mg
- Sodium: 1075 mg

## DIRECTIONS

Zest the lemon, and cut it into 8 slices. Cut the salmon into two portions, season with salt and black pepper, then spread 1 ½ tsp of pesto on each fillet. Preheat a large skillet pan with oil over medium-high flame. Add the fennel, and cook for 3 minutes or until softened and nicely golden brown. Transfer the cooked fennel to a plate, and set aside. Add the couscous and thinly sliced scallion to the pan and cook for 2 minutes or until lightly browned. Add in the olives, garlic, nuts, lemon zest, remaining pesto, and chicken broth, and stir until well combined. Add the fennel and salmon, top with lemon wedges, reduce the heat to medium-low, cover the pan, and cook for 10 to 15 minutes. Serve warm.

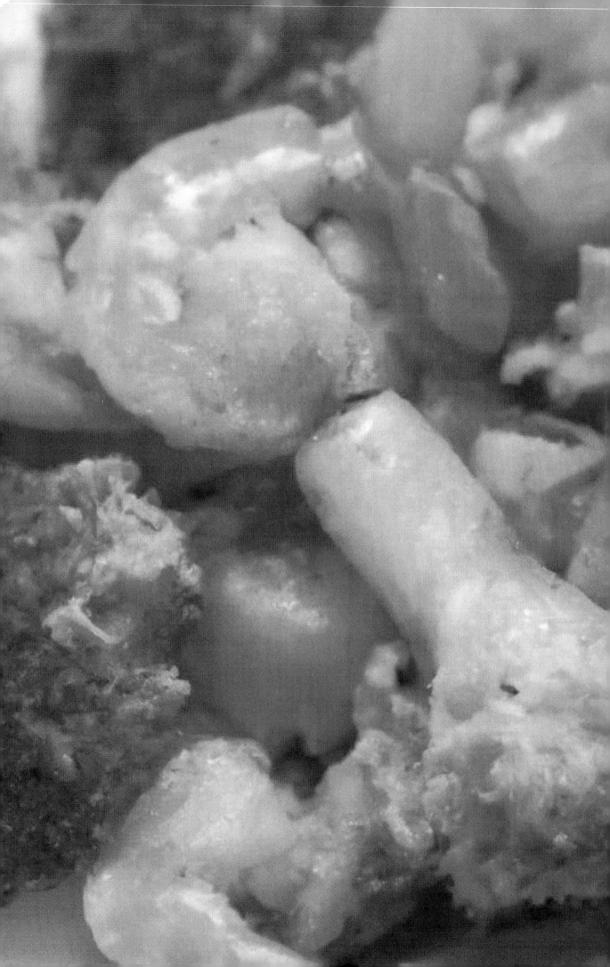

# Fish Soup

Servings: 2          Prep time: 5min          Cook time:4,30min

INGREDIENTS
1 cup of cod fillets, cubed
1 cup of medium shrimp,
peeled and deveined
1 medium white onion, peeled
and roughly chopped
½ of medium green bell
pepper, chopped
1cup of mushrooms
1cup of diced tomatoes,
¼ cup of sliced black olives
1 tsp of minced garlic
1/8 tsp of ground black
pepper
1 tsp of dried basil
3 bay leaves
1/4 tsp of fennel seed,
crushed
1/2 cup of orange juice
1/2 cup of dry white wine

DIRECTIONS
Turn on your 6-quart slow cooker on a low heat setting and place in chopped onion, green bell pepper, mushrooms, olives, garlic, black pepper, basil, bay leaves, crushed fennel seeds, orange juice, white wine, tomato sauce, 1 cup water. Stir well until mixed and combined. Shut the slow cooker with its lid and plugin, and cook for 4 to 4 hours and 30 minutes or until vegetables are tender-crisp. Then add shrimps and cod to vegetables and cook for 20 to 30 minutes or until shrimps are pink and cooked.

Nutrition:
- Calories: 509
- Fat: 6.5 g
- Fiber: 6.9 g
- Carbs: 32.4 g
- Protein: 74.7 g
- Cholesterol: 501 mg
- Sodium: 1343 mg

# Shrimp with Zucchini

Servings: 2          Prep time:40min          Cook time:15min

INGREDIENTS
1 cup of shrimp, peeled and
deveined
2 cups of zucchini, trimmed
2 tbsp of chopped fresh
parsley
2 tbsp of capers, rinsed
1 tbsp of cornstarch
1 tsp of minced garlic
salt
1/4 cup of lemon juice
1/3 cup of white wine
2 tbsp of olive oil, divided
1 cup of chicken broth

Nutrition:
- Calories: 662
- Fat: 31.4 g
- Carbs: 29.4 g
- Protein: 61.7 g
- Cholesterol: 508 mg
- Sodium: 1339 mg

DIRECTIONS
Cut zucchini into thin strips and place in a colander. Season with salt. Toss until well coated and let rest for 15 to 30 minutes to drain all juices. Meanwhile, preheat a large skillet pan with oil and garlic. Cook for 30 seconds or until fragrant and slightly softened, and then add shrimp and cook for 1 more minute. Combine the cornstarch and chicken broth in a small glass bowl and add shrimp, capers, lemon juice, and wine. Mix well and simmer for 5 more minutes or until shrimp are cooked and set aside. Drain zucchini noodles from their water and gently squeeze them to remove any excess liquid. Preheat a large skillet pan with oil over a medium-high flame and add zucchini noodles. Toss until well-coated and slightly golden brown. Cook for about 3 minutes and garnish with parsley.                    71

# Cod with Tomatoes

Servings: 2          Prep time: 10min          Cook time: 20min

## INGREDIENTS

4 skinless cod fillets,
3 cups of cherry tomatoes
2 tbsp of sliced pitted olives
2 tsp of capers
2 cloves of garlic, sliced thinly
1/4 tsp of garlic powder
salt
1/4 tsp of ground black pepper
1/4 tsp of paprika
2 tsp of fresh oregano
1 tsp of fresh thyme
1 tbsp of olive oil
1 tsp oregano leaves

Nutrition:
- Calories: 311
- Fat: 10.7 g
- Fiber: 4.5 g
- Carbs: 13.9 g
- Protein: 43 g
- Cholesterol: 110 mg
- Sodium: 894 mg

## DIRECTIONS

Preheat oven to 400F/200C. Mix the garlic powder, salt, black pepper, paprika, oregano, and thyme in a bowl, and rub half of this mixture over both sides of the cod fillets. Take a 15x10x1 inch baking pan, line it with aluminum foil, grease well with olive oil, and place seasoned cod fillets on it. Assemble tomatoes and garlic on the other side of the pan. Add oil into the remaining oregano mixture, drizzle over tomatoes, and mix until well coated.

Place the baking pan into the oven and bake for 8 to 12 minutes or until the fish is cooked, stirring tomatoes halfway through the cooking process. When baked, remove the baking pan from the oven, and stir in olives and capers into cooked tomatoes and garlic. Garnish with oregano leaves and serve while still warm.

# MEAT

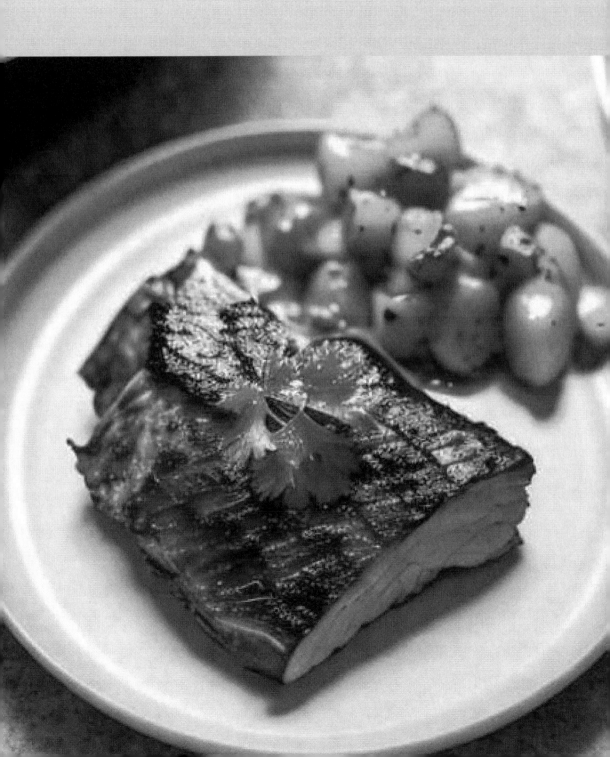

# • BEEF

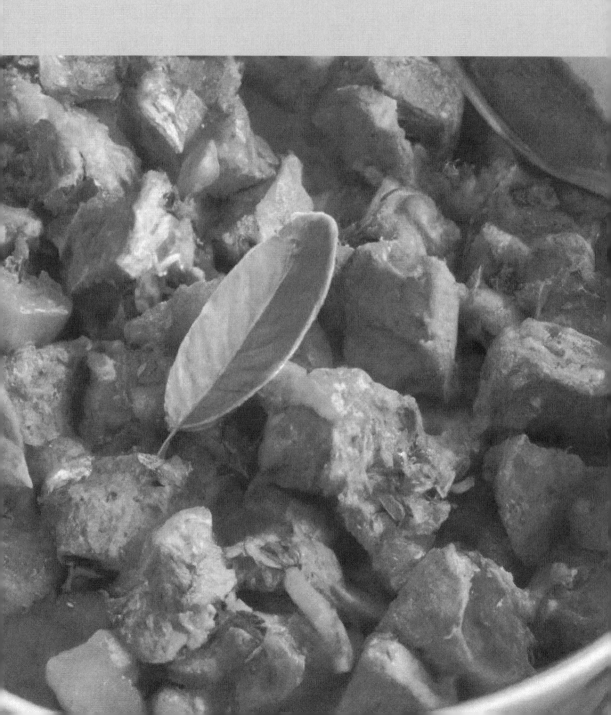

# Mexican Beef

Servings: 2          Prep time: 15min          Cook time: 20min

## INGREDIENTS

1 cup of lean ground beef
¾ cup of chopped onion
½ cup of bell pepper, any color, seeded and chopped
½ tbsp of chili powder
1 tbsp of oregano
1 cup of tomatoes, chopped
1 cup of frozen vegetable mix, chopped
2 cups of water
1/2 cup of shredded Mexican cheese blend

## DIRECTIONS

Place the beef in a large skillet and add onions. Sauté for 3 minutes or until the meat has slightly rendered its fat. Stir in the bell pepper, chili powder, and oregano, and cook for another minute. Add in the tomatoes, vegetable mix, and water. Close the lid and bring it to a simmer for 15 minutes. Before serving, stir in cheese.

Nutrition:
- Calories: 323
- Fat: 10.2 g
- Fiber: 6 g
- Carbs: 18.4 g
- Protein: 39.2 g
- Cholesterol: 108 mg
- Sodium: 174 mg

# Spicy Beef

Servings: 2          Prep time: 15min          Cook time: 40min

## INGREDIENTS

1 cup beef cut into chunks
1 medium pepper, cut into thirds
4 cloves of garlic, minced
2-inch of piece ginger, chopped
1 yellow onion, chopped
2 tbsp of ground coriander
2 tsp of ground cumin
½ tsp of ground turmeric
2 tsp of garam masala
1 tbsp of olive oil
1 cup of diced ripe tomatoes
2 cups of water
1 cup of fresh cilantro for garnish

## DIRECTIONS

In a food processor, pulse the Serrano peppers, garlic, ginger, onion, coriander, cumin, turmeric, and garam masala until well combined. Heat oil over medium flame in a skillet and sauté the spice mixture for 2 minutes or until fragrant.
Stir in the beef and cook, stirring for 3 minutes or until the meat turns brown. Stir in the tomatoes and sauté for another 3 minutes. Add the water and bring it to a boil. Once boiling, turn the heat low and simmer for thirty minutes or until the meat is tender.
Add the cilantro last before serving.

Nutrition:
- Calories 338
- Fat: 15.4 g
- Carbs: 13.8 g
- Protein: 36.8 g
- Cholesterol: 101 mg
- Sodium: 98 mg

# Beef and Pineapple

Servings: 2  Preptime:15min+mariat.   Cook time:20min

## INGREDIENTS

3/4 cup of beef shoulder steaks, cut into thick chunks

A dash of ground black pepper

2 tbsps of olive oil

2 tbsps of lime juice

2 cloves of garlic, minced

½ tsp of ground cumin

1 cup of pineapple chunks

12 skewers

Nutrition:
- Calories: 338
- Fat: 22.2 g
- Fiber: 1.3 g
- Carbs: 12.1 g
- Protein: 23.7 g
- Cholesterol: 70 mg
- Sodium: 77 mg

## DIRECTIONS

Combine the beef, black pepper, olive oil, lime juice, garlic, and cumin in a bowl until well incorporated. Place inside the fridge and allow marinating for at least 3 hours. Thread one chunk of beef and a chunk of pineapple alternately through the wooden skewer. Do two or three alternating layers. Heat the grill to 350F/176C and place the skewers on the rack. Grill for 5-10 minutes on each side.

# Beef Stew

Servings: 2          Prep time:20 min        Cook time:2,5 h

## INGREDIENTS

2 pcs lean beef casserole steak

2 cups mixed casserole veg

1 garlic bulb

1 small pack fresh thyme

1 cup long stem broccoli

Nutrition:
- Calories 362
- Fat: 3.4 g
- Carbs: 50.9 g
- Protein: 37 g
- Cholesterol: 0 mg
- Sodium: 511 mg

## DIRECTIONS

Preheat the oven to 360F/180C. Fry the cut beef into chunks in a non-stick casserole pan (suitable to put in the oven) until brown in batches. Transfer to a plate and set aside. Fray the casserole veg in the pan for about 5 minutes. Return the beef to the pan, add garlic, pour over 1 cup boiling water, and push most of the thyme under the water. Season lightly, bring to a boil, and cover. Transfer to the oven and cook for 1 ½ hours until tender. Remove the pan from the oven, and discard the thyme. Pop the garlic cloves from their skins into a bowl discarding the skins. Add a large spoonful of vegetables from the pan, puree with a stick blender, and return to the pan. Pop the pan back in over for another 30 minutes. When the stew is nearly ready, boil the broccoli until tender and drain well. Ladle the stew into shallow bowls and serve with the broccoli.

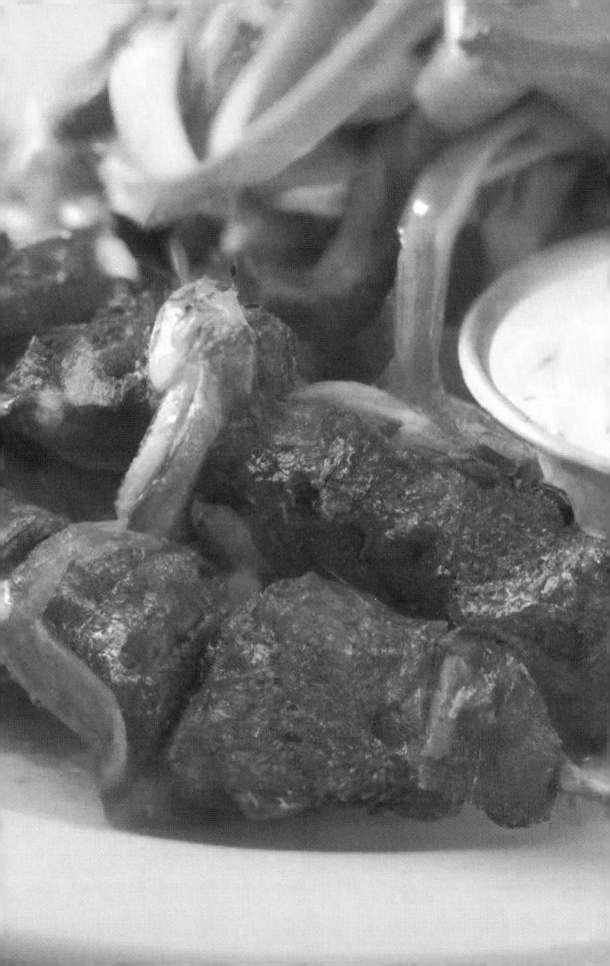

# Beef Kebab

Servings: 2    Preptime:15min+marin    Cook time:20min

## INGREDIENTS

2 large red onions

1 cup fat-free natural greek yogurt

1 tbs curry powder

2 pcs lean beef medallion steaks

2 peppers

Nutrition:
- Calories: 360
- Fat: 3.8 g
- Fiber: 4.8 g
- Carbs: 26.9 g
- Protein: 55.3 g
- Cholesterol: 3 mg
- Sodium: 28 mg

## DIRECTIONS

Roughly chop 1 onion and put it in the food processor with yogurt, add curry powder, and season lightly. Cut the beef into large chunks, add yogurt and onion to the bowl, and chill for 2 hours or overnight. Preheat the grill to high. Cut the remaining onions into large chunks and thread on the 4 skewers, marinated beef, and peppers. Arrange in a single layer on a foil-lined grill pan, season with freshly ground black pepper, and grill for 8 – 10 minutes on each side.

# Beef Zucchini Noodles

Servings: 2         Prep time:15min         Cook time:40min

## INGREDIENTS

1 cup lean beef mince, 5% fat

2 peppers

1 mixed beans in a mild chilli sauce

1 large courgette

2 tbsps Cheddar grated preheat the oven to 390F/200C

Nutrition:
- Calories 241
- Fat: 9.9 g
- Carbs: 13.3 g
- Protein: 27.8 g
- Cholesterol: 75 mg
- Sodium: 188 mg

## DIRECTIONS

Brown the beef in a nonstick pan for about 5 minutes. Then stir the peppers, beans, and chili sauce in the pan. Bring to a boil, cover, and simmer over low heat for 15 minutes. Peel the courgettes into thin ribbons using a vegetable peeler, and pat dry with kitchen paper. Tip the beef mixture into an ovenproof dish, season lightly, and arrange the courgettes in ripples to cover the beef mixture completely. Scatter over the cheese and bake for 25 minutes or until golden.

# Beef Spice Noodles

Servings: 2     Preptime:15min+marin     Cook time:15min

## INGREDIENTS

2 pcs lean beef steak

2 tbs teriyaki sauce

1 cup  dried egg noodles

1 cup mixed stir fry vegetables

1 tsp cinese five spice powder

Nutrition:
- Calories: 466
- Fat: 10.9 g
- Fiber: 3.9 g
- Carbs: 36.6 g
- Protein: 52.9 g
- Cholesterol: 156 mg
- Sodium: 1332 mg

## DIRECTIONS

Marinate the steak in teriyaki sauce for 20 minutes or longer if you have time. Cook the noodles according to the pack's instructions, drain well, rinse under cold water, and set aside. In a wok, fry the beef in batches for 2 minutes on high heat or until brown, then transfer to a bowl and keep warm. Wipe the wok, add oil, and stir-fry the vegetables for 2 minutes. Mix the five spice powders with 100 ml cold water, add to the vegetables, and bring to a boil. Return the beef to the wok, add the noodles, and stir fry for 2 minutes to heat through. Serve hot.

# Beef Pie

Servings: 2          Prep time:15min          Cook time:40min

## INGREDIENTS

1 cup beef mince

1 cup of mixed casserole veg or casserole veg pack

1 cup boiling beef stock

2 cups of potatoes

1 leek tiny slices

Nutrition:
- Calories: 649
- Fat: 15.9 g
- Carbs: 81.1 g
- Protein: 45.6 g
- Cholesterol: 134 mg
- Sodium: 1270 mg

## DIRECTIONS

Fry mince beef in a non-stick pan for 5 minutes, boil cover for another 15 minutes, then uncover and boil over high heat to reduce any liquid to a nice coating consistency. Season to taste. Boil vegetables in stock for 30 minutes. Separately cook the potatoes for 12 minutes, then at leeks and cook for 5 minutes, drain, mash, and season to taste. Preheat the grill to hot. Tip the beef mixture into an ovenproof dish, spoon over the mash to cover completely, and smooth with a fork. Grill for 3-4 minutes or until golden.

79

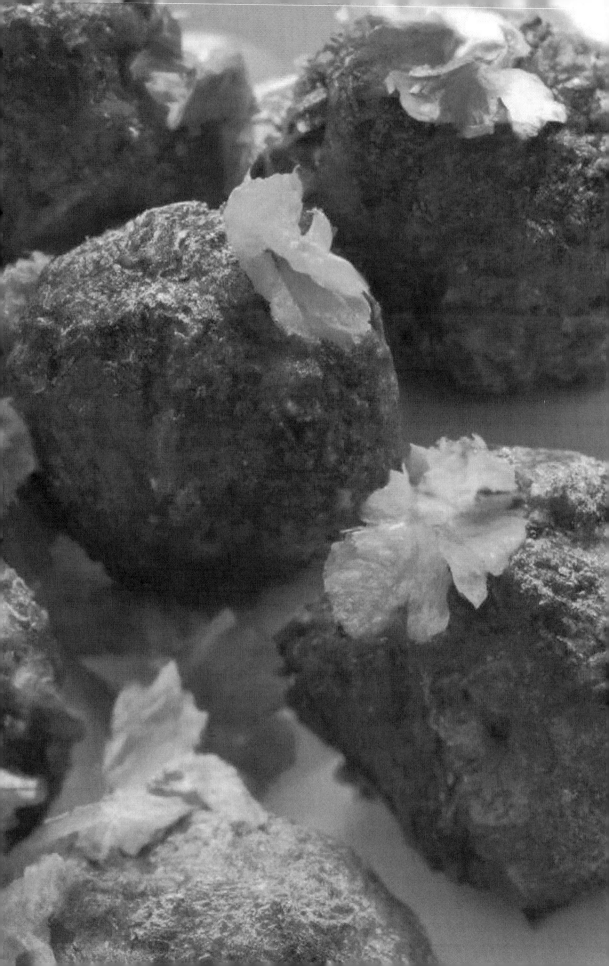

# Mushrooms Steak

Servings: 2    Preptime:15min+marin    Cook time:20min

## INGREDIENTS

2 medium sweet potatoes peeled and cut into chunks
1 cup green beans trimmed
2 pcs lean beef steaks
1/2 cup mini portobello or chestnut mushrooms
1 tbsp chopped fresh rosemary plus sprigs to garnish

Nutrition:
- Calories: 317
- Fat: 5.9 g
- Fiber: 8.7 g
- Carbs: 35.2 g
- Protein: 32.4 g
- Cholesterol: 76 mg
- Sodium: 131 mg

## DIRECTIONS

Cook the potatoes in boiling water over high heat for 12-15 minutes. Drain well, mash, and season to taste. Cook the beans for 8-10 minutes. Drain well. Fry steak and mushrooms in a nonstick pan with oil, turning them often to stop them from catching. Sprinkle over the rosemary, turn the steaks, and cook for a further 1-2 minutes or more for well done. Put mushrooms, mash, and green beans with the stake on the plate, garnish with rosemary sprigs, and serve hot.

# Beef Balls

Servings: 2    Prep time:15min    Cook time:40min

## INGREDIENTS

small pack fresh coriander roughly chopped
1 cup lean beef mince 5 % fat or less
1 tbsp tikka curry powder
1 carrot peeled an coarsely grated
1/2 cup sweetcorn with peppers from can drained and dried

## DIRECTIONS

Preheat the oven to 400F/200C.
Put most coriander in a large bowl, reserving a few chopped leaves. Add all ingredients and mix well. Divide into 12 equal-sized balls. Arrange the balls on a baking tray and bake for 25-30 minutes or until cooked through and beginning to brown. Scatter with coriander to serve

Nutrition:
- Calories: 215
- Fat: 6 g
- Carbs: 19,8 g
- Protein: 23.4 g
- Cholesterol: 62 mg
- Sodium: 131 mg

# • LAMB

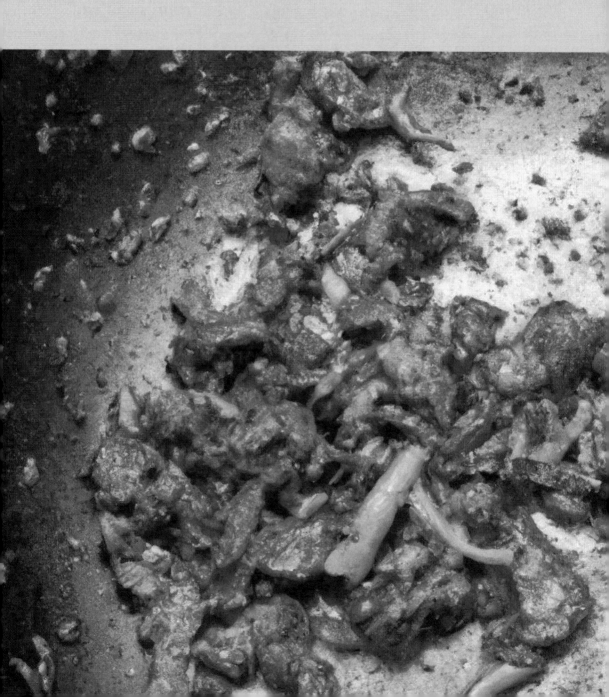

# Lamb and Sweet Potato

Servings: 2    Preptime:15min+marin    Cook time:20min

## INGREDIENTS

2 medium sweet potatoes, peeled and cut into small chunks

1 tbsp tikkacurry powder

2 red chillies 1 finely chopped and 1 sliced

4 pcs lean lamb leg steaks cut into bite size chunks

1/2 cup savoy cabbage cored and shredded

Nutrition:
- Calories: 422
- Fat: 9.5 g
- Fiber: 7.4 g
- Carbs: 44.7 g
- Protein: 38 g
- Cholesterol: 113 mg
- Sodium: 118 mg

## DIRECTIONS

Fry the potatoes in the nonstick pan for 5 minutes on medium heat until beginning to color, shaking the pan often. Sprinkle the curry powder and stir fry for 1-2 minutes. Add the chopped chilli and pour over 150 ml of boiling water. Bring to a boil over high heat, cover, and cook for 7-8 minutes or until tender. Drain tip into a bowl and keep warm. Use the liquid as a sauce if you like. Fry the lamb for 5 – 8 minutes in a nonstick pan or until browned, then scatter over the cabbage and cook for 5 minutes, stirring frequently. Return the sweet potatoes to the pan and stir fry for 1 minute more to heat through. Season to taste, scatter over the sliced chilli and serve hot.

# Lamb with Chilli Greens

Servings: 2    Prep time:15min    Cook time:40min

## INGREDIENTS

1 inc piece fresh root ginger

2 large garlic cloves crushed

2 large lean lamb leg steaks

1 large red chillies deseeded and chopped

1 cup spring greens sliced

Nutrition:
- Calories: 623
- Fat: 24.2 g
- Carbs: 2.8 g
- Protein: 92.1 g
- Cholesterol: 294 mg
- Sodium: 250 mg

## DIRECTIONS

Cut half of the ginger into matchstick and grate the rest. Add grated ginger, 1 garlic clove crushed, and a little seasoning in a bowl. Stir, add the lamb steaks, and coat well. Cover and marinate for 15 minutes. Fry the lamb in a nonstick griddle pan on high heat for 2 ½ minutes on each side or until nicely charred on both sides. Lift onto a plate cover and leave to rest for 5 minutes.

Meanwhile, in a nonstick pan over high heat, stir the ginger, matchsticks remaining garlic, and most of the chilli for 40 seconds. Add the spring greens and 3 tbsp water and stir-fry for 3 -4 minutes. Divide the greens and steaks between plates and serve hot with the remaining chilli.    83

# Lamb Kebabs

Servings: 2    Preptime: 15min + marin    Cook time: 20min

## INGREDIENTS

2 lemons

1 tsp sweet paprika

2 pcs  lean lamb leg steaks

2 peppers

1 medium courgette sliced

Nutrition:
- Calories: 253
- Fat: 9.5 g
- Fiber: 2 g
- Carbs: 6.1 g
- Protein: 35.9 g
- Cholesterol: 113 mg
- Sodium: 97 mg

## DIRECTIONS

Finely grate the zest, squeeze the juice from 1 lemon into a bowl, and stir in the paprika and a little seasoning. Cut the lamb into bite-size chunks, add to the bowl, and mix to coat well. Cover and marinate for a few hours. Preheat the grill to medium. Cut the remaining lemons into thin wedges and thread on onto 4 metal skewers along with the lamb peppers and courgettes. Leave a little space between the lamb so it can cook evenly. Arrange the skewers in a single layer on a foil-lined grill pan and grill for 15-20 minutes or until cooked to your liking turning frequently.

# Lamb's Livers

Servings: 2  Preptime: 10min    Cook time: 40min

## INGREDIENTS

1 cup green beans trimmed

2 cups parsnips peeled and

cut into chunks

a few fresh sage leaves, sliced

1 large onion, thinly sliced

1 cup lambs liver

Nutrition:
- Calories 420
- Fat: 6 g
- Carbs: 68.4 g
- Protein: 25.6 g
- Cholesterol: 0 mg
- Sodium: 34 mg

## DIRECTIONS

Rinse liver under cold running water, and slice thickly. Cover and set aside. On medium heat, fry onions for 8 – 10 minutes or until nicely colored. Add sage, pour with 250 ml boiling water, and simmer over low heat for 15 minutes or until the onion is soft. Puree a little of the mixture with a stick blender and set aside. Cook the parsnips in boiling water for 10-12 minutes or until tender. Drain well, mash, season to taste, and keep warm. Cook the green beans for 3-4 minutes or until just tender. Drain well. Keep warm. In a large nonstick pan, warm the oil and add liver. Fry over high heat on each side of the liver for 2-3 minutes, add onion sauce, and bubble for another few minutes until the liver is tender. Serve with mash and green beans.

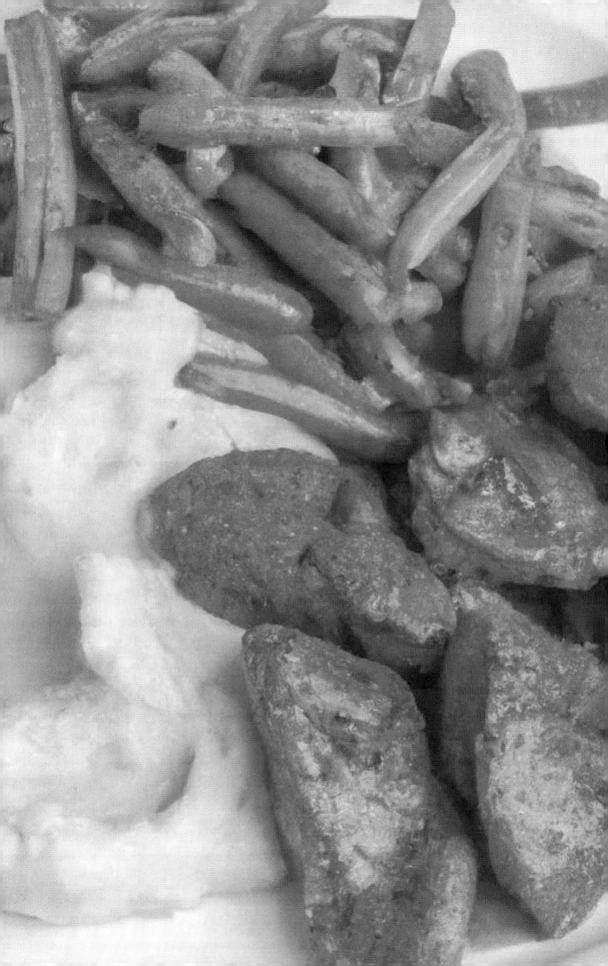

# Roast Lamb

Servings: 2    Preptime:15min                Cook time:30min

## INGREDIENTS

4 pcs of French-style lamb rib roast, trimmed from fat
1 cup of dry red wine
2 cloves of garlic, minced
1 tsp of freshly grated nutmeg
1 tbsp of olive oil
1 tbsp of chopped rosemary
3 tbsps of dried cranberries, chopped

Nutrition:
- Calories: 475
- Fat: 24.6 g
- Fiber: 1.4 g
- Carbs: 6.7 g
- Protein: 33.8 g
- Cholesterol: 112 mg
- Sodium: 111 mg

## DIRECTIONS

In a resealable plastic, place the lamb and add red wine, garlic, nutmeg, olive oil, and rosemary. Seal the bag and turn it to coat the lamb with the spices. Marinate inside the fridge for at least 4 hours while turning the bag occasionally. Preheat the oven to 375F/190C. Remove the lamb from the marinade. Reserve the juices. Place the lamb bone side down on a roasting pan lined with foil. Pour the reserved marinade over the roasting pan. Roast for 30 minutes until the lamb turns slightly golden. Turn the lamb every 10 minutes and baste it with the sauce. Once cooked, take out the lamb from the oven and slice. Serve with chopped cranberries on top.

# Cumin Lamb

Servings: 2        Prep time:10min            Cook time:25min

## INGREDIENTS

1 tbsp of olive oil
1 red onion, chopped
1 cup of cherry tomatoes, halved
1 cup lamb stew meat, ground
1 tbsp of chili powder
Black pepper to the taste
2 tsps of cumin, ground
1 cup of low-sodium veggie stock
2 tbsps of cilantro, chopped

Nutrition:
- Calories 324
- Fat: 16.2 g
- Carb: 11.2 g
- Protein: 33.9 g
- Cholesterol: 102 mg
- Sodium: 156 mg

## DIRECTIONS

Heat the pan with the oil over a medium-high flame. Add the onion, lamb, and chili powder, toss, and cook for 10 minutes. Add the rest of the ingredients, toss, and cook over medium heat for 15 minutes more. Divide into bowls and serve.

# Fennel Lamb

Servings: 2     Preptime:10min          Cook time:40min

INGREDIENTS

1 cup of lamb shoulder, boneless and cubed
8 white mushrooms, halved
2 tbsps of olive oil
1 yellow onion, chopped
2 garlic cloves, minced
1 and ½ tbsps of fennel powder
Black pepper to the taste
A bunch of scallions, chopped
1 cup of low-sodium veggie stock

DIRECTIONS

Heat a pan with the oil over medium flame. Add the onion and the garlic, and cook for 5 minutes. Add the meat and the mushrooms, mix, and cook for 5 minutes more. Add the other ingredients, mix, bring to a simmer, and cook over medium heat for 30 minutes. Divide the mix into bowls and serve.

Nutrition:
- Calories: 379
- Fat: 22.7 g
- Fiber: 2.3 g
- Carbs: 9.6 g
- Protein: 35.3 g
- Cholesterol: 102 mg
- Sodium: 252 mg

# Lamb and Radishes

Servings: 2     Prep time:10min         Cook time:35min

INGREDIENTS

½ cup of low-sodium veggie stock
1 cup of lamb stew meat, cubed
1 cup of radishes, cubed
1 tbsp of cocoa powder
Black pepper to the taste
1 yellow onion, chopped
1 tbsp of olive oil
2 garlic cloves, minced
1 tbsp of parsley, chopped

DIRECTIONS

Heat a pan with the oil over medium-high fire; add the onion and the garlic, and sauté for 5 minutes. Add the meat and cook until brown for 2 minutes on each side.
Add the stock and the other ingredients; bring to a simmer, and cook over medium heat for 25 minutes more. Divide everything between plates and serve.

Nutrition:
- Calories: 318
- Fat: 15.8 g
- Carbs: 10 g
- Protein: 34.6 g
- Cholesterol: 102 mg
- Sodium: 241 mg

# Lamb in Mustard Sauce

Servings: 2   Preptime:30min                    Cook time:20min

## INGREDIENTS

1/3 cup of light cream
2/3 cup of beef stock
1 tbsp of mustard
2 tsp of Worcestershire sauce
1 cup of lamb chops
2 tbsp of olive oil
1 tbsp of fresh rosemary chopped
2 garlic cloves; minced
2 tbsp of ghee
A spring of rosemary
A spring of thyme
1 tbsp of shallot; chopped.
2 tsp of lemon juice
black pepper

Nutrition:
- Calories: 556
- Fat: 44.5 g
- Fiber: 1.6 g
- Carbs: 4.8 g
- Protein: 34.7 g
- Cholesterol: 162 mg
- Sodium: 412 mg

## DIRECTIONS

Mix 1 tbsp of oil with garlic, salt, pepper, and rosemary in a bowl and whisk well. Add the lamb chops to coat and leave aside for a few minutes. Heat a pan with the rest of the oil over medium-high fire; add lamb chops, reduce heat to medium, cook them for 7 minutes, flip, cook them for 7 minutes more, transfer to a plate, and keep them warm. Return the pan to medium heat; add shallots, stir, and cook for 3 minutes. Add the stock, stir, and cook for 1 minute. Add the Worcestershire sauce, mustard, cream, rosemary, and thyme spring; stir and cook for 8 minutes. Add the lemon juice, salt, pepper, and ghee; discard rosemary and thyme; mix well and remove the heat. Serve lamb with sauce.

# Lamb and Mint

Servings: 2        Prep time:10min              Cook time:8,3h

## INGREDIENTS

2 pcs of lamb leg

6 mint leaves

1 tbsp of maple extract

2 tbsps of mustard

1/4 cup of olive oil

1 tsp of garlic; minced

A pinch of rosemary; dried

4 thyme spring

Salt and black pepper,

Nutrition:
- Calories: 552
- Fat: 11.8 g
- Carbs: 5.7 g
- Protein: 23.2 g
- Cholesterol: 80 mg
- Sodium: 70 mg

## DIRECTIONS

Put the oil in your slow cooker. Add the lamb, salt, pepper, maple extract, mustard, rosemary, and garlic; rub well, cover, and cook on Low for 7 hours. Add the mint and thyme and cook for 1 more hour. Leave the lamb to cool down a bit before slicing and serving with pan juices on top.

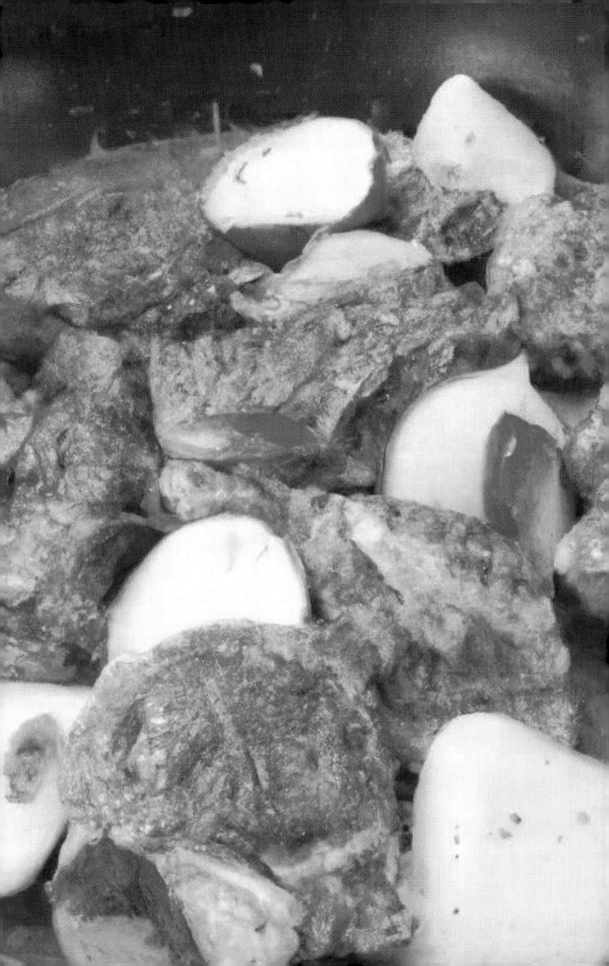

# • PORK

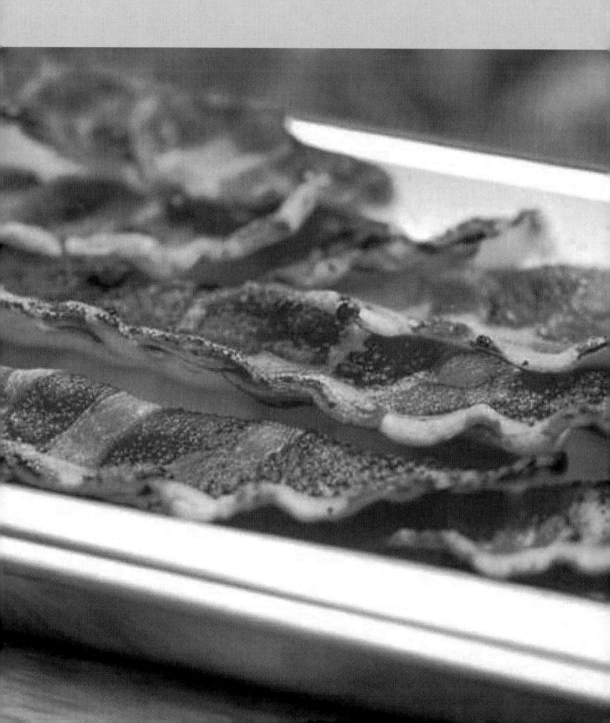

# Pork with Apples

Servings: 2    Preptime:15min                Cook time:30min

## INGREDIENTS

1 cup of apple cider
2 tbsps of maple syrup
¼ tsp of smoked paprika powder
1 tsp of grated ginger
¼ tsp of ground black pepper
2 tsp of olive oil
1 1/2 cups of pork tenderloin
1 large sweet potato, cut into cubes
1 large apple, cored and into cubes

Nutrition:
- Calories: 468
- Fat: 9.7 g
- Fiber: 6.0 g
- Carbs: 59.4 g
- Protein: 37.7 g
- Cholesterol: 93 mg
- Sodium: 113 mg

## DIRECTIONS

Preheat the oven to 375F/190C. Combine the apple cider, maple syrup, smoked paprika, ginger, and black pepper in a bowl. Set aside. Heat the oil in a large skillet and sear the meat for 3 minutes on both sides. Transfer the pork to a baking dish and place the sweet potatoes and apples around the pork. Pour in the apple cider sauce. Place inside the oven and cook for 20 minutes.

# Pork and Garlic

Servings: 2    Prep time:10min                Cook time:45 min

## INGREDIENTS

1 cup of pork meat, boneless and cubed
1 red onion, chopped
1 tbsp of olive oil
3 garlic of cloves, minced
1 cup of low-sodium beef stock
2 tbsps of sweet paprika
Black pepper to the taste
1 tbsp of chives, chopped

Nutrition:
- Calories: 418
- Fat: 24.4 g
- Carbs: 27.3 g
- Protein: 23.8 g
- Cholesterol: 80 mg
- Sodium: 190 mg

## DIRECTIONS

Heat a pan with the oil over medium flame. Add the onion and the meat, toss, and brown for 5 minutes. Add the remaining ingredients, toss, reduce heat to medium, cover, and cook for 40 minutes. Divide the mix between plates and serve.

# Pork and Carrots

Servings: 2    Preptime:10min            Cook time:30min

## INGREDIENTS

1 cup of pork stew meat, cubed
¼ cup of low-sodium veggie stock
2 carrots, peeled and sliced
2 tbsps of olive oil
1 red onion, sliced
2 tsp of sweet paprika
Black pepper

## DIRECTIONS

Heat a pan with the oil over medium flame; add the onion, stir, and sauté for 5 minutes. Add the meat, toss, and brown for 5 minutes more. Add the rest of the ingredients, simmer, and cook over medium heat for 20 minutes. Divide the mix between plates and serve.

Nutrition:
- Calories: 415
- Fat: 25.5 g
- Fiber: 3.5 g
- Carbs: 12.5 g
- Protein: 34.7 g
- Cholesterol: 98 mg
- Sodium: 221 mg

# Pork with Cumin

Servings: 2        Prep time:10min            Cook time:45 min

## INGREDIENTS

½ cup of low-sodium stock
2 tbsps of olive oil
1 cup of pork stew meat, cubed
1 tsp of coriander, ground
2 tsp of cumin, ground
Black pepper to the taste
1 cup of cherry tomatoes, halved
4 garlic cloves, minced
1 tbsp of cilantro, chopped

## DIRECTIONS

Heat a pan with the oil over medium flame. Add the garlic and the meat, toss, and brown for 5 minutes. Add the stock and the other ingredients. Bring to a simmer and cook over medium heat for 40 minutes. Divide between plates and serve.

Nutrition:
- Calories 432
- Fat: 27.4 g
- Carbs: 6.7 g
- Protein: 36.7 g
- Cholesterol: 98 mg
- Sodium: 176 mg

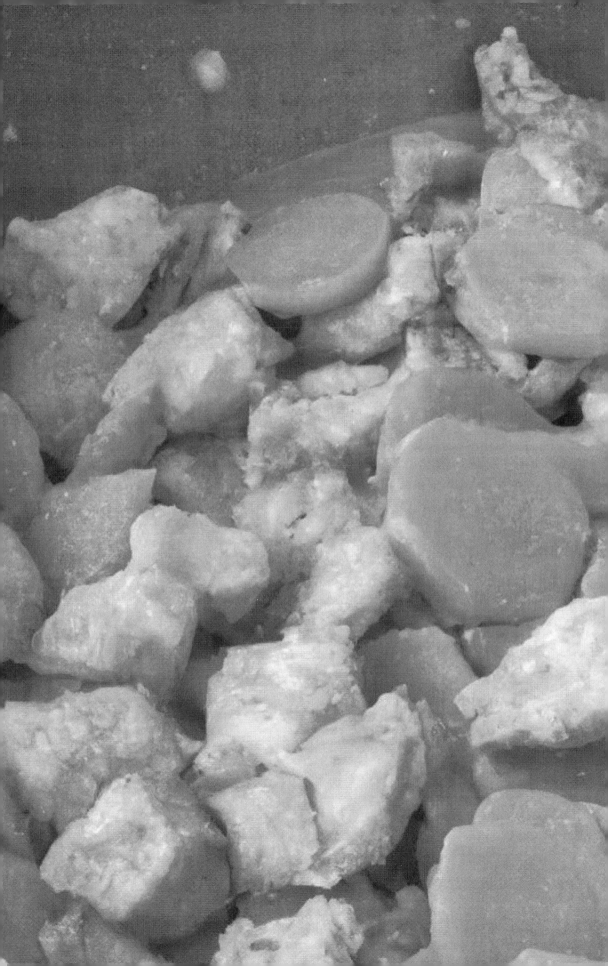

# Pork and Greens

INGREDIENTS

2 tbsps of balsamic vinegar
1/3 cup of coconut aminos
1 tbsp of olive oil
1 cup of mixed salad greens
1 cup of cherry tomatoes, halved
1 cup of pork stew meat, cut into strips
1 tbsp of chives, chopped

DIRECTIONS

Heat a pan with the oil over medium flame. Add the pork, aminos, and vinegar, toss, and cook for 15 minutes.

Add the salad greens and the other ingredients, toss, cook for 5 minutes more, divide between plates, and serve.

Nutrition:
- Calories: 217
- Fat: 12.2 g
- Fiber: 1.6 g
- Carbs: 12.7 g
- Protein: 12 g
- Cholesterol: 0 mg
- Sodium: 80 mg

# Spiced Pork

INGREDIENTS

3 tbsps of olive oil
1 pcs of pork shoulder roast
2 tsp of sweet paprika
1 tsp of garlic powder
1 tsp of onion powder
1 tsp of nutmeg, ground
1 tsp of allspice, ground
Black pepper to the taste
1 cup of low-sodium veggie stock

DIRECTIONS

In your slow cooker, combine the roast with the oil and the other ingredients, toss, put the lid on, and cook on low for 8 hours. Slice the roast, divide it between plates, and serve with the cooking juices drizzled on top.

Nutrition:
- Calories: 498
- Fat: 51.4 g
- Carbs: 4.9 g
- Protein: 20.7 g
- Cholesterol: 80 mg
- Sodium: 546 mg

# Pork and Zucchini

## INGREDIENTS

1 cup of pork loin boneless, trimmed and cubed

2 tbsp of avocado oil

¾ cup of low-sodium veggie stock

½ tbsp of garlic powder

1 tbsp of marjoram, chopped

2 zucchinis, roughly cubed

1 tsp of sweet paprika

Black pepper to the taste

## DIRECTIONS

Heat a pan with the oil over a medium-high flame. Add the meat, garlic powder, and marjoram, toss and cook for 10 minutes. Add the zucchini and the other ingredients, toss, bring to a simmer, reduce heat to medium, and cook the mix for 20 minutes more. Divide everything between plates and serve.

Nutrition:
- Calories: 404
- Fat: 27.5 g
- Fiber: 3.9 g
- Carbs: 10.4 g
- Protein: 33.7 g
- Cholesterol: 120 mg
- Sodium: 472 mg

# Pork and Tomatoes

Servings: 2          Prep time:10min          Cook time:30min

## INGREDIENTS

2 garlic cloves, minced

1 cup of pork stew meat, ground

2 cups of cherry tomatoes, halved

1 tbsp of olive oil

Black pepper to the taste

1 red onion, chopped

½ cup of low-sodium veggie stock

2 tbsp of low-sodium tomato paste

1 tbsp of parsley, chopped

## DIRECTIONS

Heat a pan with the oil over medium flame; add the onion and the garlic, toss, and sauté for 5 minutes. Add the meat and brown it for 5 minutes more. Add the rest of the ingredients, toss, bring to a simmer, cook over medium heat for 20 minutes more, divide into bowls, and serve.

Nutrition:
- Calories: 369
- Fat: 19.4 g
- Carbs: 14.4 g
- Protein: 36.7 g
- Cholesterol: 98 mg
- Sodium: 739 mg

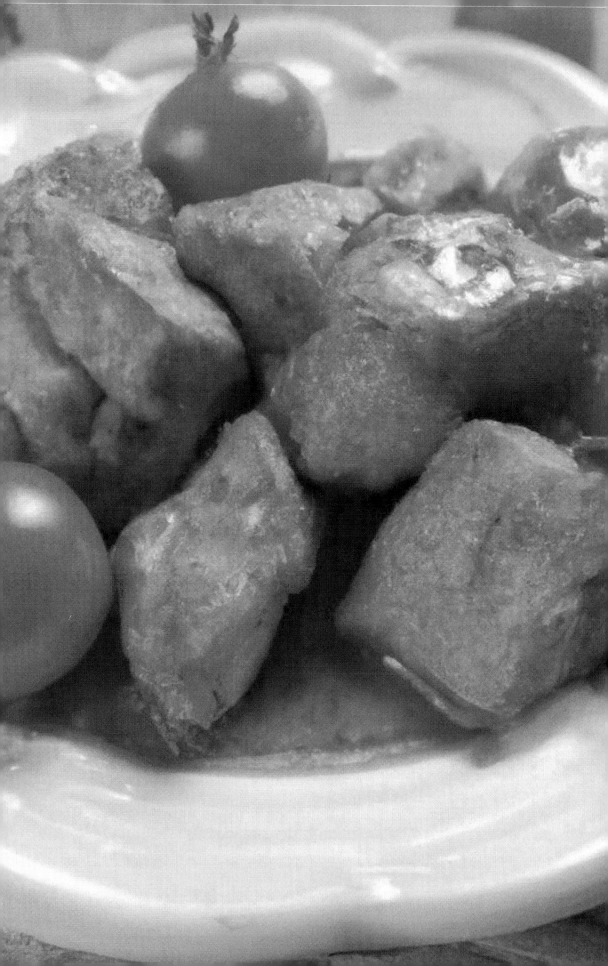

# Sage Pork Chops

Servings: 2     Preptime:10min          Cook time:35min

## INGREDIENTS

1/2 pound pork chops

2 tbsp of olive oil

1 tsp of smoked paprika

1 tbsp of sage, chopped

2 garlic cloves, minced

1 tbsp of lemon juice

Black pepper to the taste

## DIRECTIONS

In a baking dish, combine the pork chops with the oil and the other ingredients, toss, introduce in the oven, and bake at 400F/200C for 35 minutes. Divide the pork chops between plates and serve with a side salad.

Nutrition:
- Calories: 474
- Fat: 37.5 g
- Fiber: 0.9 g
- Carbs: 4.4 g
- Protein: 33.5 g
- Cholesterol: 60 mg
- Sodium: 3 mg

# Pesto Pork

Servings: 2     Prep time:10min          Cook time:40min

## INGREDIENTS

2 tbsp of olive oil

2 spring onions, chopped

1/2 pound of pork chops

2 tbsp of basil pesto

1 cup of cherry tomatoes, cubed

2 tbsp of low-sodium tomato paste

½ cup of parsley, chopped

½ cup of low-sodium veggie stock

Black pepper to the taste

## DIRECTIONS

Heat a pan with the olive oil over a medium-high flame. Add the spring onions and the pork chops, and brown for 3 minutes on each side. Add the pesto and the other ingredients, toss gently, bring to a simmer, and cook over medium heat for 30 minutes more. Divide everything between plates and serve.

Nutrition:
- Calories: 542
- Fat: 43 g
- Carbs: 13.4 g
- Protein: 28.1 g
- Cholesterol: 98 mg
- Sodium: 295 mg

# Pork and Spinach Pan

Servings: 2    Preptime:10min    Cook time:30min

## INGREDIENTS

1 cup of pork, ground
2 tbsp of olive oil
1 red onion, chopped
1 cup of baby spinach
4 garlic cloves, minced
½ cup of low-sodium
veggie stock
½ cup of canned tomatoes,
chopped
Black pepper to the taste
1 tbsp of chives,
chopped

Nutrition:
- Calories: 792
- Fat: 62.5 g
- Fiber: 15.3 g
- Carbs: 23.9 g
- Protein: 37.2 g
- Cholesterol: 0 mg
- Sodium: 53 mg

## DIRECTIONS

Heat a pan with the oil over a medium-high flame. Add the onion and the garlic, toss, and cook for 5 minutes. Add the meat, toss, and brown for 5 minutes more. Add the remaining ingredients except the spinach, toss, bring to a simmer, reduce heat to medium, and cook for 15 minutes. Add the spinach, toss, cook the mix for another 5 minutes, divide everything into bowls, and serve.

# Pork with Avocados

Servings: 2    Prep time:10min    Cook time:15min

## INGREDIENTS

2 cups of baby spinach
1/2 pound of pork steak,
cut into strips
1 tbsp of olive oil
1 cup of cherry tomatoes,
halved
2 avocados, peeled, pitted
and cut into wedges
1 tbsp of balsamic vinegar
½ cup of low-sodium veggie
stock

Nutrition:
- Calories 662
- Fat: 31.4 g
- Carbs: 29.4 g
- Protein: 61.7 g
- Cholesterol: 508mg
- Sodium: 1339 mg

## DIRECTIONS

Heat a pan with the oil over a medium-high flame. Add the meat, toss, and cook for 10 minutes. Add the spinach and the other ingredients, toss, cook for 5 minutes more, divide into bowls, and serve.

98

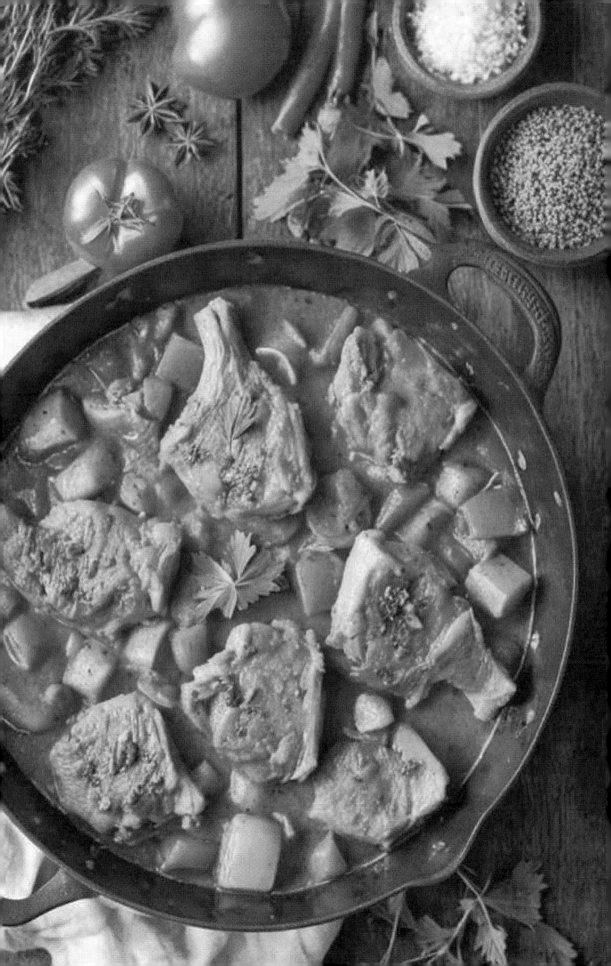

# • CHICKEN

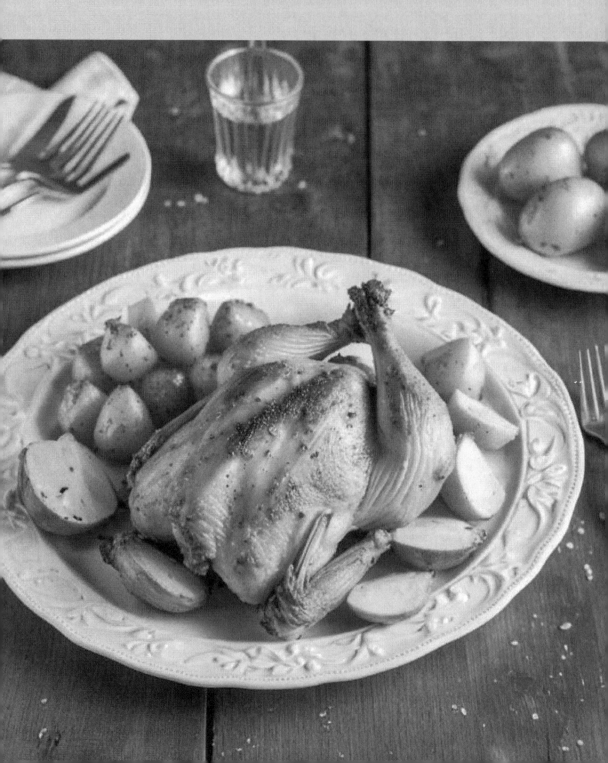

# Chicken and Spinach

Servings: 2      Prep time: 10min      Cook time: 20min

## INGREDIENTS

2 tbsps of olive oil
2 chicken breasts, skinless and boneless
A pinch of black pepper
1 tbsp of low-fat butter
1/2 tbsp of oregano, dried
3 garlic cloves, minced
2 cups of baby spinach
1 cup of canned artichokes, no-salt-added, chopped
1/2 cup of roasted red peppers, chopped
1/2 cup of coconut cream
1/2 cup of low-fat mozzarella, shredded
2 tbsps of parmesan, grated

## DIRECTIONS

Heat a pan with the oil over a medium-high flame. Add chicken, season with black pepper and oregano, cook for 8 minutes on each side, and transfer to a bowl. Heat the same pan with the butter over a medium-high flame. Add garlic, spinach, artichokes, and red peppers, stir, and cook for 3 minutes. Return chicken breasts, add mozzarella, parmesan, and coconut cream, toss, bring to a simmer, cook for 8 minutes more, divide into bowls, and serve.

Nutrition:
- Calories: 600
- Fat: 44 g
- Fiber: 7 g
- Carbs: 19 g
- Protein: 38 g
- Cholesterol: 103 mg
- Sodium: 507 mg

# Chicken Onion Mix

Servings: 2      Prep time: 10min      Cook time: 30min

## INGREDIENTS

3 tbsps of olive oil
1 yellow onion, roughly chopped
2 tsps of thyme, chopped
2 garlic cloves, minced
A pinch of black pepper
2 chicken breasts, skinless, boneless, and cubed
1/2 tbsp of oregano, dried
3/4 cup of low-sodium beef stock
1 tbsp of parsley, chopped

## DIRECTIONS

Heat a pan with 2 tbsp of olive oil over medium-low flame. Add the onion, black pepper, and thyme, toss and cook for 2 minutes. Add garlic, cook for 1 more minute, and transfer to a bowl. Clean the pan, and heat it with the rest of the oil over a medium-high fire. Add chicken, black pepper, and oregano, stir and cook for 10 minutes. Add the beef stock, add the onion mix and the parsley, toss, cook for 15 minutes, divide into bowls, and serve.

Nutrition:
- Calories: 325
- Fat: 23 g
- Carbs: 7 g
- Protein: 22 g
- Cholesterol: 64 mg
- Sodium: 55 mg

# Asian Chicken

Servings: 2      Prep time:10min                    Cook time:30min

## INGREDIENTS

4 chicken thighs, boneless and
skinless
1/4 cup of coconut aminos
1/4 cup of balsamic vinegar
3 tbsps of garlic, minced
1/4 cup of olive oil
A pinch of black pepper
1 tbsp of green onion, chopped
3 tbsps of garlic chili sauce

Nutrition:
- Calories: 397
- Fat: 29g
- Fiber: 0.3g
- Carbs: 9.7 g
- Protein: 22.9g
- Cholesterol 95mg
- Sodium 132mg

## DIRECTIONS

Put the oil in a baking dish, add chicken, aminos, vinegar, garlic, black pepper, onion, and chili sauce, toss well, put in the oven, and bake at 425F/220C for 30 minutes. Divide the chicken and the sauce between plates and serve.

# Chicken  Veggie

Servings: 2            Prep time:10min                    Cook time:25min

## INGREDIENTS

2 chicken breasts, skinless,
boneless, and cubed
2 tbsps of olive oil
½ tsp of Italian seasoning
A pinch of black pepper
½ cup of yellow onion,
chopped
1 cup chopped tomatoes,
1 cup of cauliflower florets

## DIRECTIONS

Heat a pan with the oil over a medium-high flame. Add chicken, black pepper, onion, and Italian seasoning, toss and cook for 5 minutes. Add the tomatoes and cauliflower, toss, cover the pan, and cook over medium heat for 20 minutes. Toss again, divide everything between plates, and serve.

Nutrition:
- Calories 291
- Fat: 17.4g
- Carbs: 9g
- Protein: 25.8g
- Cholesterol 73mg
- Sodium 78mg

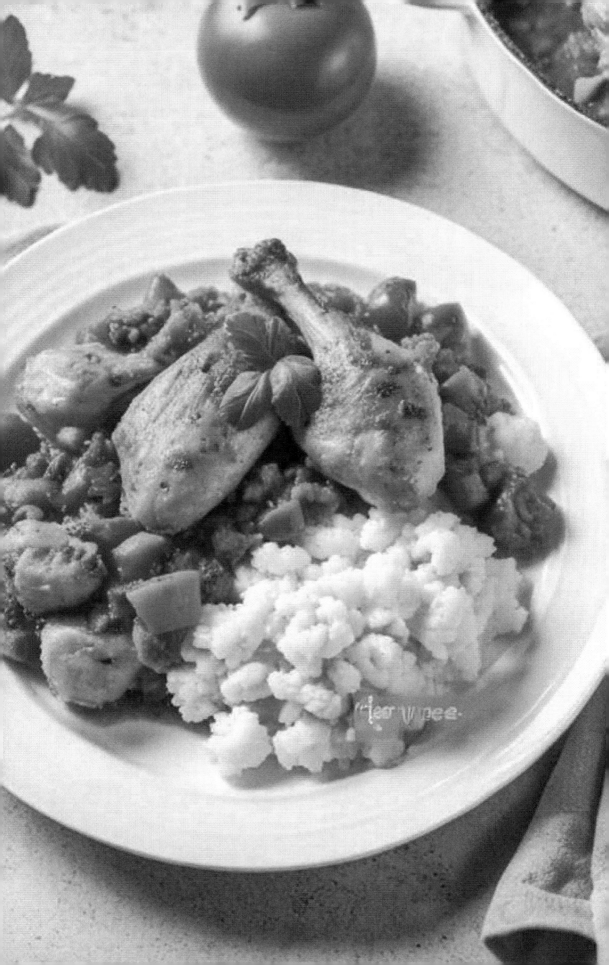

# Chicken and Black Beans

Servings: 2    Prep time: 10min          Cook time: 25min

INGREDIENTS

1 cup of chicken breasts, skinless and boneless
1 cup of water
1 tbsp of olive oil
1/2 cup of coconut milk
1/2 cup of pumpkin flesh
1/2 cup of canned black beans, no-salt-added, drained and rinsed
1 tbsp of cilantro, chopped

Nutrition:
- Calories: 509
- Fat: 27.2g
- Fiber: 9.4g
- Carbs: 36.6g
- Protein: 32.6g
- Cholesterol 62mg
- Sodium 76mg

DIRECTIONS

Heat a pan with the oil over a medium-high flame. Add the chicken and fry until meat is brown on each side. Add the water, milk, pumpkin, and black beans, toss, cover the pan, reduce heat to medium, and cook for 20 minutes. Add the cilantro, toss, divide between plates, and serve.

# Chicken Sweet Potato

Servings: 2    Prep time: 10min          Cook time: 30min

INGREDIENTS

2 chicken breasts, skinless, boneless, and cubed
1 yellow onion, chopped
2 tbsps of olive oil
1 garlic clove, minced
4 sweet potatoes, cubed
2 carrots, chopped
½ tbsp of ginger, grated
½ tbsp of cumin, ground
A pinch of black pepper
2 cups veggie stock

Nutrition:
- Calories 494
- Fat: 19.5g
- Carbs: 57.1g
- Protein: 27.6g
- Cholesterol 72mg
- Sodium 838mg

DIRECTIONS

Heat a pot with the oil over a medium-high flame. Add onion and garlic, stir, and cook for 5 minutes. Add the carrots and potatoes, stir, and cook for 5 minutes. Add the ginger, cumin, stock, pepper, and chicken. Stir, boil, reduce heat to medium, simmer for 20 minutes, ladle into soup bowls, and serve.

# Coconut Chicken

Servings: 2    Prep time:10min    Cook time:50min

## INGREDIENTS

3 tbsps of olive oil
4 chicken thighs
A pinch of salt and black pepper
3 garlic cloves, minced
1 cup of mushrooms, halved
1/2 cup of coconut cream
½ tsp of basil, dried
½ tsp of oregano, dried
1 tbsp of mustard

## DIRECTIONS

Heat a pot with 2 tbsp of oil over a medium-high flame. Add chicken, salt, and pepper, brown for 3 minutes on each side, and transfer to a plate. Heat the same pot with the rest of the oil over medium fire. Add mushroom and garlic, stir, and cook for 6 minutes. Add the salt, pepper, oregano, basil, and chicken, mix and bake in the oven at 400F/200C for 30 minutes. Add the cream and mustard, stir, bake for 10 minutes, divide everything between plates, and serve.

Nutrition:
- Calories: 490
- Fat: 41.6g
- Fiber: 2.7g
- Carbs: 8.2g
- Protein: 26.2g
- Cholesterol: 95mg
- Sodium: 112mg

# Chicken Cili

Servings: 2    Prep time:10min    Cook time:70min

## INGREDIENTS
1/2 cup of coconut flour
6 lemon tea bags
a pinch of salt
a pinch of black pepper
1 cup of chicken breast, skinless, boneless, and cubed
4 tbsps of olive oil
1 cup of celery, chopped
3 garlic cloves, minced
1 yellow onion, chopped
1 red bell pepper, chopped
1/2 cup of Poblano pepper, chopped
1 cup veggie stock
1 tsp of chili powder
¼ cup of cilantro, chopped

## DIRECTIONS
Dredge the chicken pieces in coconut flour. Heat a pot with the oil over a medium-high flame. Add chicken, cook for 5 minutes on each side, and transfer to a bowl. Heat the pot again over a medium-high fire. Add onion, celery, garlic, bell pepper, and Poblano pepper, stir, and cook for 2 minutes. Add the stock, chili powder, salt, pepper, chicken, and tea bags, stir, bring to a simmer, reduce heat to medium-low, cover, and cook for 1 hour. Discard tea bags, add cilantro, stir, ladle into bowls, and serve.

Nutrition:
- Calories: 688
- Fat: 38.4 g
- Carbs: 58g
- Protein: 34.5g
- Cholesterol: 72mg
- Sodium: 479mg

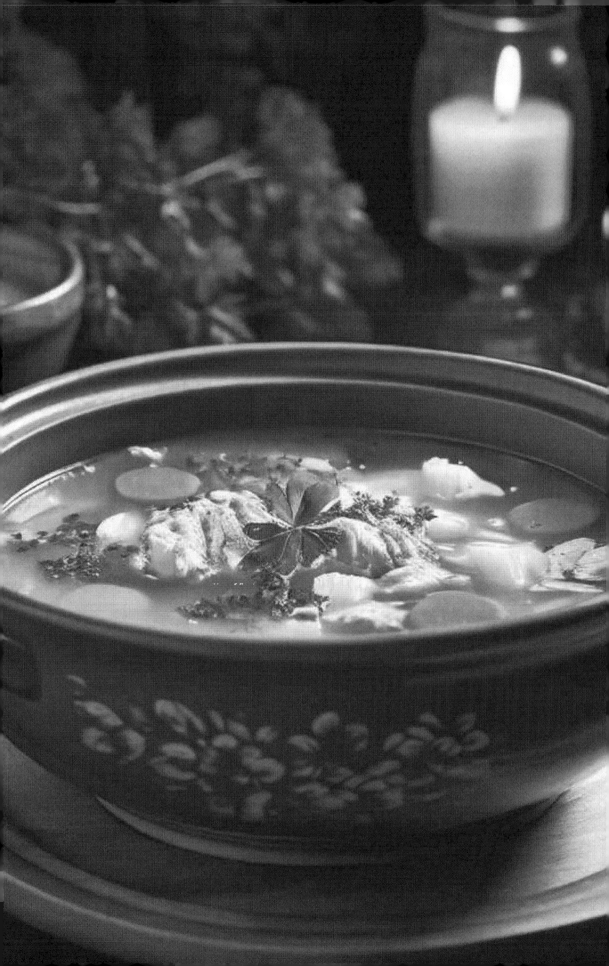

# Chicken Casserole

Servings: 2    Prep time:10min    Cook time:40min

## INGREDIENTS

1 tbsp of oil
1 white onion, chopped
2 cloves of garlic, minced
1 cup cooked turkey meat, shredded
1 tbsp rosemary
1 zucchini, chopped
1 carrot, peeled and chopped
½ cup water
Pepper to taste

## DIRECTIONS

Preheat oven to 400F/200C. Grease an oven-safe casserole dish with oil. Mix the onion, garlic, turkey, pepper, salt, and rosemary in a bowl. Pour into prepared casserole dish. Sprinkle carrot on top, followed by zucchini, and then pour water over the mixture. Cover the dish with foil and bake for 25 minutes or until bubbly hot. Remove foil, return to oven, and broil the top for 2 minutes on high. Let it rest for 10 minutes.

Nutrition:
- Calories: 239
- Fat: 10.8g
- Fiber: 3.8g
- Carbs: 13.5 g
- Protein: 22.8g
- Cholesterol: 53mg
- Sodium: 85mg

# Chicken Soup

Servings: 2    Prep time:10min    Cook time:30min

## INGREDIENTS

1/2 chicken,
1 cup of coconut milk
1 cup of water
1 tbsp fresh cilantro, chopped
1 tbsp of ginger
1 tbsp of cumin
1 tbsp of coriander
½ tsp of salt
½ tsp of curry
1 lemon, juice extracted

## DIRECTIONS

Place a heavy-bottomed pot on a medium-high fire. Add all the ingredients except for coconut milk. Mix well. Bring to a boil. Once boiling, lower the fire to a simmer and cook for 20 minutes. Stir in coconut milk. Continue simmering for another 10 minutes.

Nutrition:
- Calories: 364
- Fat: 30.9g
- Carbs: 12.9g
- Protein: 14.5g
- Cholesterol: 32mg
- Sodium: 635mg

# Chicken Meatloaf

Servings: 2    Prep time: 10min            Cook time: 35min

## INGREDIENTS

pinch of salt
1/8 tbsp of pepper
2 eggs
¼ cup of parsley, chopped
¼ cup of coconut flakes
½ tbsp of jalapeno, seeded and diced
½ cups of diced mango
1 cup of yellow bell pepper, diced
1 cup of ground chicken
1 tbsp of oil

Nutrition:
- Calories: 339
- Fat: 20.1g
- Fiber: 2.8g
- Carbs: 13.4g
- Protein: 27.4g
- Cholesterol: 226mg
- Sodium: 208mg

## DIRECTIONS

Preheat oven to 400F/200C and lightly grease a loaf pan with oil. In a large bowl, mix all the ingredients. Evenly spread in a prepared pan and cover the pan with foil. Pop in the oven and bake for 30 minutes. Remove foil and broil the top for 3 minutes. Let it sit for 10 minutes.

# Chicken with Mushrooms

Servings: 2    Prep time: 10min            Cook time: 25min

## INGREDIENTS

2 tbsps of chopped fresh parsley
4 slices Muenster cheese
1 garlic clove, minced
1 cup of sliced fresh mushrooms
1 cup of water
1 cup of creamy mushroom soup,
1 chicken breast, sliced thinly
¼ tbsp of pepper
2 tbsps of all-purpose flour

Nutrition:
- Calories: 363
- Fat: 22 g
- Carbs: 13g
- Protein: 28.2g
- Cholesterol: 90mg
- Sodium: 777mg

## DIRECTIONS

Place a nonstick saucepan on medium-high heat for 3 minutes. Add the oil and swirl the pan to coat the sides and bottom with oil. Heat for a few seconds. Add the chicken and sauté until no longer pink, around 5 minutes. Season with pepper and transfer to a plate. In the same pan, add flour and sauté for 3 minutes. Add garlic and sauté for a minute more. Stir in mushrooms and cook for 5 minutes until water comes from it. Add the remaining ingredients, except for cheese and parsley. Mix well. Return chicken to pan. Let chicken absorb for 1 minute. Add cheese just for 1 min. Put on a plate and sparkle with parsley.

# Chicken and Pineapple

Servings: 2    Preptime: 10min                Cook time: 30min

INGREDIENTS

2 tbsps of cornstarch

1 small yellow bell pepper, cut

1 small red bell pepper, cut

1 can of pineapple chunks, drained and ¼ cup liquid set aside

1 cup of BBQ sauce

2 cloves of garlic, chopped finely

4 pcs of boneless, skinless chicken thighs

1 tbsp of oil

Nutrition:
- Calories: 412
- Fat: 13g
- Fiber: 4.6g
- Carbs: 48g
- Protein: 22g
- Cholesterol: 88mg
- Sodium: 520mg

DIRECTIONS

Place a heavy-bottomed pot on medium-high fire and heat the pot for 3 minutes. Once hot, add oil and stir around to coat the pot with oil. Add the chicken and cook for 4 minutes per side. Meanwhile, in a bowl, mix the cornstarch with ¼ cup water and set aside. Add the pineapple chunks to the pot and sauté for 2 minutes. Stir in and add the liquid from pineapple, BBQ sauce, and garlic. Mix well and bring to a boil. Cover and lower the fire, and simmer for 8 minutes. Stir in bell peppers and cornstarch slurry. Continue mixing and cooking until the sauce has thickened, around 5 minutes.

# Sesame Chicken

Servings: 2    Prep time: 10min                Cook time: 20min

INGREDIENTS

1 tbsp of toasted sesame seeds

2 green onions, chopped

3 tbsps of water

2 tbsps of cornstarch

¼ tbsp of red pepper flakes

2 tbsps of honey

2 tbsps of sesame oil

1 tbsp ketchup

2 tbsps of soy sauce

2 garlic cloves, minced

½ cup of onion, diced

1 tbsp of olive oil

Pepper to taste

2 medium boneless, skinless chicken breasts, chopped in cubes

DIRECTIONS

Place a heavy-bottomed pot on medium-high fire and heat for 3 minutes. Meanwhile, season the chicken generously with pepper. Once hot, add oil and stir around to coat the pot with oil. Stir in the garlic and onion. Cook for 3 minutes. Add the chicken and cook for 5 minutes. Stir in the red pepper flakes, ketchup, and soy sauce. Mix well. Cover, boil, lower the fire, and simmer for 5 minutes. Meanwhile, in a bowl, mix cornstarch with water and set aside. Stir in honey, sesame seeds, and sesame oil. Pour the cornstarch slurry and continue mixing while cooking until the sauce has thickened.

Nutrition:
- Calories: 613
- Fat: 27.6g
- Carbs: 86.5g
- Protein: 12.8g
- Cholesterol: 48mg
- Sodium: 1029mg

# • TURKEY

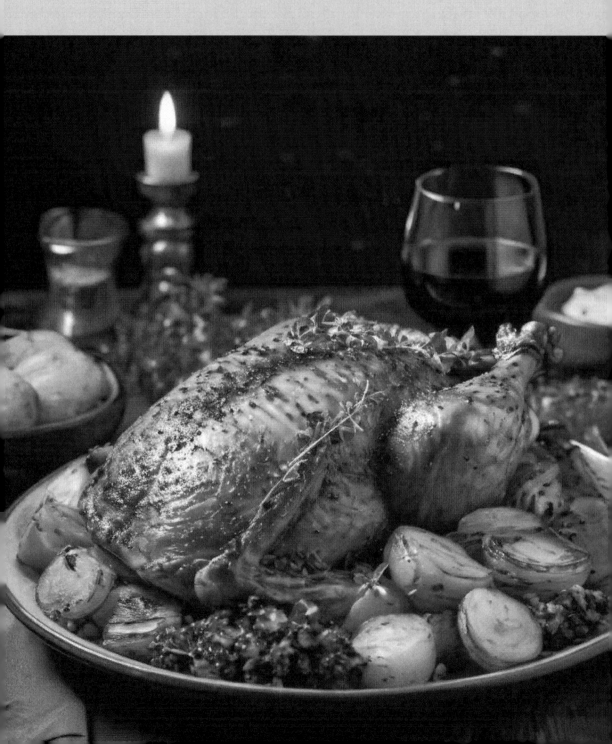

# Zucchini Turkey

Servings: 2     Prep time:10min            Cook time:40min

## INGREDIENTS

1 tbsp of oil
1 white onion, chopped
2 cloves of garlic, minced
1 cup cooked turkey meat, shredded
1 tbsp of rosemary
1 zucchini, chopped
1 carrot, peeled and chopped
½ cup water
Pepper to taste

Nutrition:
- Calories: 239
- Fat: 10.8g
- Fiber: 3.8g
- Carbs: 13.5g
- Protein: 22.8g
- Cholesterol: 53mg
- Sodium: 85mg

## DIRECTIONS

Preheat oven to 400F/200C. Grease an oven-safe casserole dish with oil. Mix the onion, garlic, turkey, pepper, salt, and rosemary in a bowl. Pour into prepared casserole dish. Sprinkle carrot on top, followed by zucchini, and then pour water over the mixture. Cover the dish with foil and bake for 25 minutes or until bubbly hot. Remove foil, return to oven, and grill the top for 2 minutes on high. Let it rest for 10 minutes before serving.

# Turkey Legs

Servings: 2     Prep time:10min            Cook time:30min

## INGREDIENTS

4 turkey legs
1/2 cup of light coconut milk
1 cup of water
1 ½ tbsp of lemon juice
¼ cup of cilantro, chopped
Pepper to taste

## DIRECTIONS

Place a heavy-bottomed pot on a medium-high fire. Add all the ingredients except for coconut milk. Mix well. Bring to a boil. Once boiling, lower the fire to a simmer and cook for 20 minutes. Stir in the coconut milk. Continue simmering for another 10 minutes.

Nutrition:
- Calories: 443
- Fat: 28g
- Carbs: 3.7g
- Protein: 43.3g
- Cholesterol: 163mg
- Sodium: 181mg

# Turkey with Chili

Servings: 2     Prep time:10min     Cook time:25min

## INGREDIENTS

1 tbsp of olive oil
1 cup of ground turkey
1 onion, chopped
1 green bell pepper, seeded and chopped
3 carrots, peeled and chopped
2 stalks of celery, sliced thinly
1 cup of chopped tomatoes
3 Poblano chilies, chopped
½ cup of water
3 tbsps of chili powder
1 ½ tsp of ground cumin
Pepper to taste

## DIRECTIONS

Place a heavy-bottomed pot on medium-high fire and heat for 3 minutes. Add the oil; swirl to coat the bottom and sides of the pot and heat for a minute. Stir in the turkey. Brown and crumble for 8 minutes. Season generously with pepper. Discard excess fat. Add all the ingredients. Mix well. Bring to a boil. Once boiling, lower the fire to a simmer and cook for 15 minutes.

Nutrition:
- Calories: 349
- Fat: 16.7g
- Fiber: 9.6g
- Carbs: 29.5g
- Protein: 26.5g
- Cholesterol: 65mg
- Sodium: 283mg

# Turkey Saltimbocca

Servings: 2     Prep time:5min     Cook time:15min

## INGREDIENTS

2 thin cut turkey steaks
2 parma ham slices
3 large fresh sage leaves
3/4 cup boiling chicken stock
1 cup mangetout

Nutrition:
- Calories: 183
- Fat: 3.3g
- Carbs: 5.5g
- Protein: 32.5g
- Cholesterol: 16mg
- Sodium: 616mg

## DIRECTIONS

Season the meat with freshly ground black pepper. Probably you will not need salt as ham is salty. Arrange a slice of ham and a sage leaf on top of each turkey's steak and secure it with sticks. In a nonstick pan, cook the meat on medium-high heat on each side until it is brown all around. Pour over the stock and cook for 10-15 minutes. Lift the turkey steaks onto a hot plate, remove the sticks, and cover to keep warm. Increase the heat and add the mangetout to the stock. Cook rapidly for 1-2 minutes or until the mangetout are hot, and the stock has thickened a little. Divide the vegetable between plates and top with the turkey. Pour the sauce into a jug to serve with turkey.

112

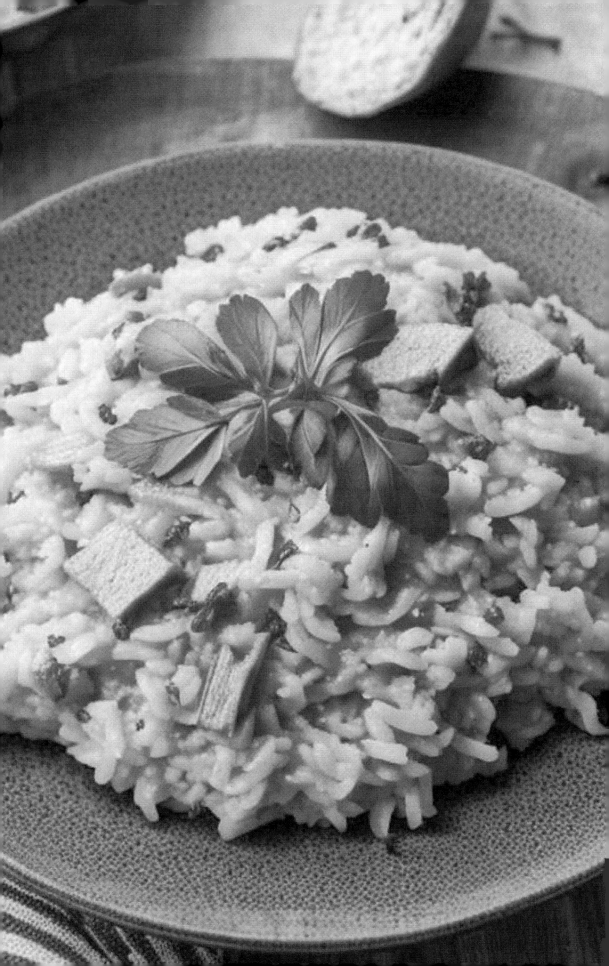

# Turkey Jalfrezi

Servings: 2    Prep time:10min    Cook time:35min

## INGREDIENTS

1 large red onion cut into chunks

2 peppers deseeded and cut into chunks

2 tsp mild curry powder

1 cup lean turkey mince 5 % fat

1 cup chopped tomatoes

2 cloves of garlic

Nutrition:
- Calories: 146
- Fat: 3.6g
- Fiber: 5.4g
- Carbs: 18.2g
- Protein: 13g
- Cholesterol: 0mg
- Sodium: 13mg

## DIRECTIONS

Place the pan over medium heat. Add the onion, garlic, and peppers and stir fry for 2 minutes, then add the curry powder and cook for 1 minute. Add the turkey and stir fry for 5 minutes breaking up the mince. Tip in the chopped tomatoes. Season lightly, cover, and simmer over low heat for 20 minutes. Stir occasionally and add water if necessary. Uncover and simmer for about 5 minutes to thicken the sauce to your liking. Serve hot.

# Turkey with Leeks

Servings: 2    Prep time:5min    Cook time:30min

## INGREDIENTS

2 skinless and boneless turkey breasts

1 leek thinly sliced

1 tsp fresh thyme leaves plus springs to garnish

1/2 cup natural fromage frais

2 level tbsp freshly grated Parmesan cheese

Nutrition:
- Calories: 233
- Fat: 7g
- Carbs: 14.6g
- Protein: 28.1g
- Cholesterol: 61mg
- Sodium: 1257mg

## DIRECTIONS

Preheat oven to 400F/200C. Season the meat and bake in the oven for 20-25 minutes or until cooked, turning halfway. Meanwhile, cook the leeks thyme and 1/2 cup boiling water in a pan over medium heat for 10-12 minutes or until the leeks have softened and most of the liquid has gone, occasionally stirring (add a little more water if needed). Reduce the heat to as low as possible, stir in the fromage frais and most of the Parmesan, and cook for 1-2 minutes or until just heated through, stirring often. Season to taste. Spoon the creamy leeks into shallow bowls and top with the chicken. Sprinkle with the remaining Parmesan and garnish with thyme springs to serve.

# Turkey Risotto

Servings: 2     Prep time:5min                    Cook time:35min

INGREDIENTS

2 large skinless and boneless
turkey breasts
1 cup dried risotto rice
2 cups boiling chicken stock
1 leek, thinly sliced
2 level tbsp freshly grated
Parmesan cheese

Nutrition:
- Calories: 600
- Fat: 7.2g
- Fiber: 2g
- Carbs: 81g
- Protein: 48g
- Cholesterol: 90mg
- Sodium: 639mg

DIRECTIONS

Cut the chicken into bite-size chunks, add to the nonstick hot pan, and fry for 5 minutes or until beginning to brown on high heat. Reduce the heat to medium-low and add the rice and $\frac{1}{4}$ of the stock. Simmer for 10 minutes, stirring frequently, and add more stock for a lovely creamy texture. Stir in the leeks and simmer for 10-15 minutes or until the rice is just cooked and most of the stock has been absorbed, stirring frequently. Sprinkle over the cheese and black pepper, and serve hot.

# Turkey and Kale Bake

Servings: 2          Prep time:10min            Cook time:1h

INGREDIENTS

2 cups potatoes halved
lengthways
1 large garlic bulb, cloves
separated
1 lemon grated zest and juice
6 skinless and boneless turkey
thighs
1/2 cup kale shredded

Nutrition:
- Calories: 269
- Fat: 6g
- Carbs: 28g
- Protein: 25g
- Cholesterol: 90mg
- Sodium: 1409 mg

DIRECTIONS

Cook the potatoes in boiling water over high heat. Drain well and tip into a roasting tin. Peel and finely grate 3 garlic cloves, mix with half of the lemon zest and lemon juice and rub into Turkey to coat. Season lightly, slash the flesh of each thigh a few times, and arrange it on top of the potatoes. Tuck the garlic cloves around and cook in the oven for 20 minutes. Scatter kale over the turkey and cook for 15 minutes or until the kale is crispy and the meat is cooked. Scatter the remaining lemon zest to serve.

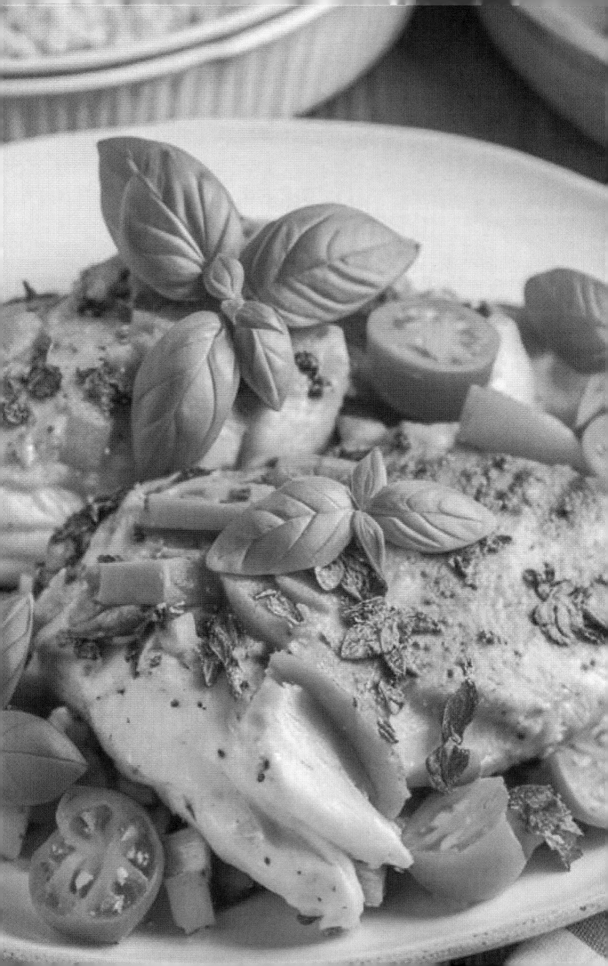

# Turkey Sandwich

Servings: 2       Prep time:10min           Cook time:0min

## INGREDIENTS

1 cup diced celery

1/2 cup finely chopped red onion

4 cups cooked turkey, diced

1 tbsp parsley, chopped,

1 tbsp lemon juice,

1/2 cup mayonnaise,

1/8 tsp ground black pepper

salt,

8 to 12 slices bread,

lettuce leaves

## DIRECTIONS

Combine the celery, red onion, turkey, and parsley in a large bowl. Toss to blend the ingredients. Combine the lemon juice, mayonnaise, and black pepper separately. Stir the liquid in the turkey mixture until blended, and add salt to taste. Line slices of bread with lettuce leaves and fill with the turkey mixture. Top with the second piece of bread. Cut in half and serve.

Nutrition:
* Calories: 709
* Fat: 25g
* Fiber: 2.4g
* Carbs: 30 g
* Protein: 85.8g
* Cholesterol: 220mg
* Sodium: 694mg

# Turkey Cutlets

Servings: 2          Prep time:15min           Cook time:25min

## INGREDIENTS

4 turkey breast cutlets

salt,

ground black pepper,

1/4 cup all-purpose flour

1/4 cup soft breadcrumbs

1/4 cup grated cheese

1 tbsp coarsely chopped fresh parsley, more for garnish

1 tsp dried basil

1 tbsp spicy brown mustard

1 large egg

1 tbsp oil

## DIRECTIONS

Lightly sprinkle both sides of the cutlets with salt and pepper and set aside. Put the flour on a pie plate and set aside. In a food processor, pulse the breadcrumbs, grated cheese, parsley, and basil until the mixture forms fine crumbs. Pour the mixture into a pie plate. In another bowl, whisk together the mustard and egg. Dip the cutlets in the flour to coat, followed by the egg mixture, and last in the breadcrumb mixture. Place the bread cutlets in the oiled baking pan and bake for 20 to 25 min at 360F/180C.

Nutrition:
* Calories: 626
* Fat: 23g
* Carbs: 23g
* Protein: 80g
* Cholesterol: 223mg
* Sodium: 1052mg

# Turkey Meatloaf

Servings: 2      Prep time:10min                Cook time:40min

## INGREDIENTS

1 large egg
1 tbsp milk
1/4 cup breadcrumbs
1/3 cup ketchup, divided
1 tsp Worcestershire sauce
2 garlic cloves minced
1/3 cup finely chopped onion
salt
1/2 tsp ground black pepper
1/2 cup ground turkey

Nutrition:
- Calories: 203
- Fat: 5g
- Fiber: 2.3g
- Carbs: 24 g
- Protein: 16.2g
- Cholesterol: 109mg
- Sodium: 1214mg

## DIRECTIONS

Preheat the oven to 350F/176C. In a large bowl, combine the egg, milk, breadcrumbs, 2 tsp ketchup, Worcestershire sauce, garlic powder, onion powder, salt, and pepper. Mix to blend thoroughly. Add the ground turkey. Gently knead the mixture together until just combined. Transfer the turkey meatloaf to the baking nonstick rack and form a loaf. Spread the remaining ketchup over the meatloaf. Bake for 40 min. Remove from the oven, and let it rest for 10 minutes before transferring it to a platter and slicing.

# Turkey with Cheese

Servings: 2      Prep time:20min                Cook time:35min

## INGREDIENTS

2 Turkey breasts
1 cup shredded mozzarella cheese
1/2 cup all-purpose flour
1 large egg
3/4 cups breadcrumbs
1/4 cup Parmesan cheese,
Salt, to taste
Pepper, to taste
1/4 cup olive oil
1 cup marinara sauce
1/2 cup mozzarella cheese, sliced
Chopped parsley for garnish

## DIRECTIONS

Preheat the oven to 400F/200C. Split the breasts with a knife. Be careful not to cut all the way through. Stuff the center with half of the shredded mozzarella. Fold the top half of the chicken over the top of the mozzarella stuffing. If it is too full, take a little cheese out. Toss some salt and pepper with the flour in a shallow bowl. Beat the egg with salt and pepper in another shallow bowl. Toss the breadcrumbs with Parmesan cheese in a third shallow bowl. Dip the stuffed breast into the flour, then flip to coat both sides in the flour mixture, dip into the egg mixture and flip to coat both sides. The last breadcrumbs cover both sides thickly.

Continue to the next page                    118

# Turkey with Cheese

Servings: 2    Prep time                    Cook time

DIRECTIONS

Continuous from the previous page

Heat the olive oil in a large oven-proof skillet. Add the cutlets so that they fit snugly but not overlapping. Fry on both sides until golden brown; they do not have to be cooked. Add the marinara sauce around the outside of the cutlets and a little on the top of each cutlet. Top the cutlets with fresh mozzarella. Place in the preheated oven and bake for about 20 minutes. Serve with chopped parsley.

Nutrition:
- Calories 1124
- Fat: 63g
- Carbs: 76g
- Protein: 64.7g
- Cholesterol: 230g
- Sodium 2720mg

# Turkey with Rice

Servings: 2        Prep time:10min        Cook time:15min

INGREDIENTS

1 tsp olive oil
1 onion, finely chopped
1½ tsp garam masala
2 garlic cloves, crushed
1 cup brown rice
1 cup roast turkey, shredded
1/2 lemon juice,
1/2 lemon wedges to serve
1 1/2 cup baby leaf spinach
Large bunch of fresh coriander, chopped
Natural yogurt to serve

Nutrition:
- Calories: 510
- Fat: 8g
- Carbs: 82g
- Protein: 26g
- Cholesterol: 50mg
- Sodium: 918mg

DIRECTIONS
Boil the rice as indicated on the package, drain well, and set aside. Heat the oil in a large frying pan and fry the onion for 5 minutes until softening. Add the garam masala and garlic and fry for 1-2 minutes more. Add the rice and turkey with a splash of water and warm for a couple of minutes, then squeeze in the lemon juice and stir in the spinach in 2 batches, letting the first wilt so you can fit it all in the pan. Add most of the coriander and stir in well. Taste, season, and sprinkle with the remaining coriander, then serve with lemon wedges and yogurt.

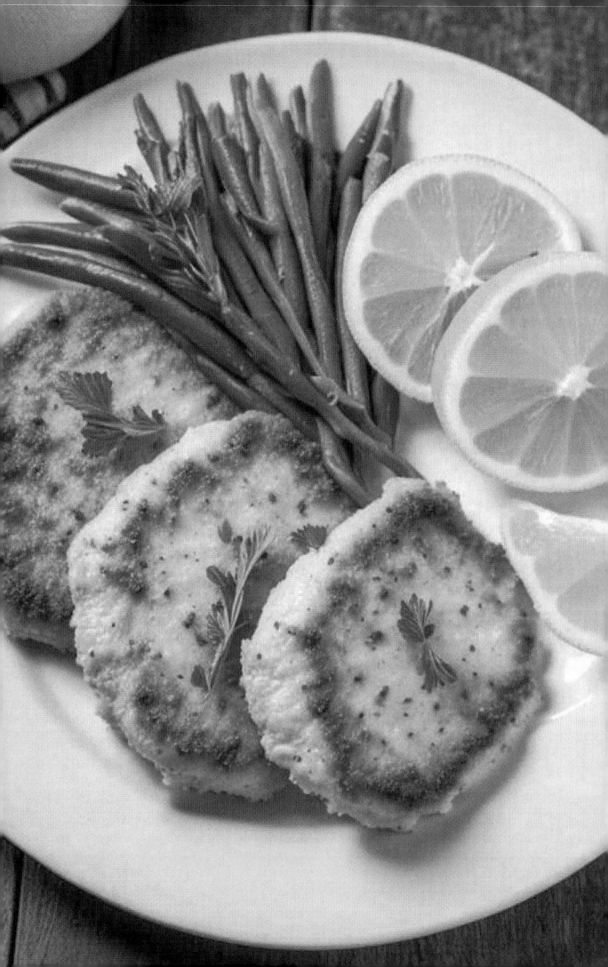

# VEGETABLES

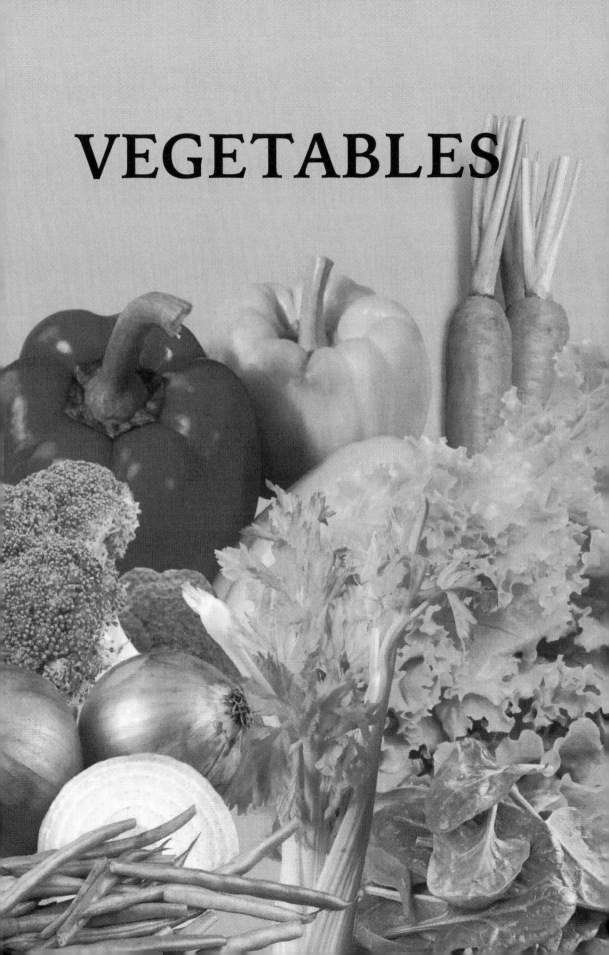

# Beans Side Dish

Servings: 2    Prep time:10min    Cook time:0min

## INGREDIENTS

1/2 cup canned kidney beans, drained and rinsed

1/2 cup canned garbanzo beans, drained

1/2 cup canned pinto beans, drained

3 tbsps balsamic vinegar

2 tbsps olive oil

2 tbsps garlic powder

1 small onion diced

## DIRECTIONS

In a large salad bowl, combine the beans with vinegar, oil, seasoning, garlic powder, and onion, toss, divide between plates, and serve as a side dish.

Nutrition:
- Calories: 643
- Fat: 18.1g
- Fiber: 23.4g
- Carbs: 91.9g
- Protein: 30g
- Cholesterol: 0mg
- Sodium: 26mg

# Cucumber Mix

Servings: 2    Prep time:10min    Cook time:0min

## INGREDIENTS

1 big cucumber, peeled and chopped

1 small red onion, chopped

4 tbsps of non-fat yogurt

1 tsp of balsamic vinegar

## DIRECTIONS

Mix the onion with cucumber, yogurt, and vinegar in a bowl. Toss, divide between plates, and serve as a side dish.

Nutrition:
- Calories: 69
- Fat: 0.2g
- Carbs: 14.3g
- Protein: 2.8g
- Cholesterol: 1mg
- Sodium: 30mg

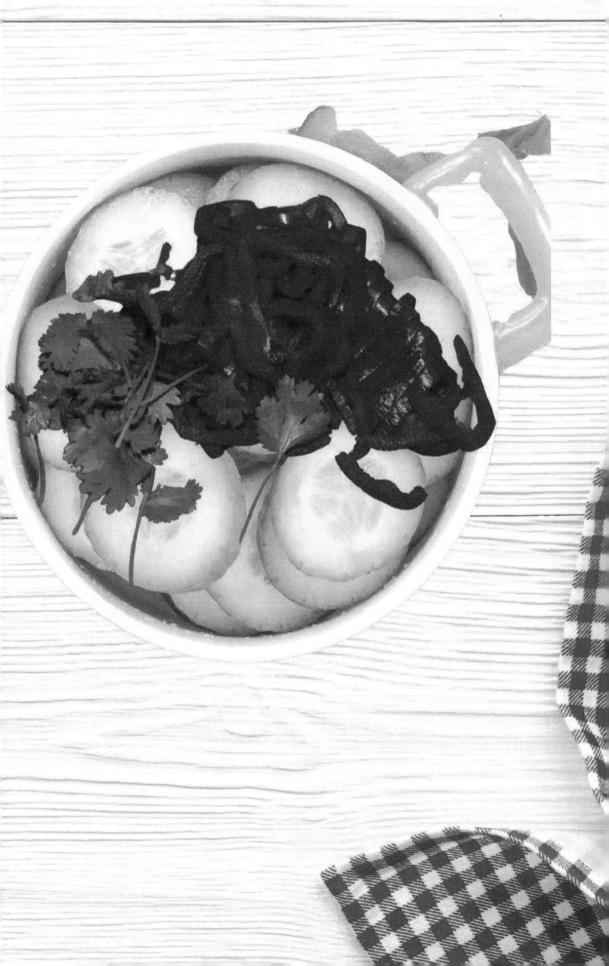

# Peppers Mix

Servings: 2    Prep time:10min    Cook time:10min

### INGREDIENTS

1 tbsp olive oil
2 tbsps garlic powder
2 red bell peppers, chopped
2 yellow bell peppers, chopped
2 orange bell peppers, chopped
Black pepper to the taste

### DIRECTIONS

Heat a pan with the oil over a medium-high flame. Add all the bell peppers, stir, and cook for 5 minutes. Add garlic powder and black pepper, stir, cook for 5 minutes, divide between plates, and serve as a side dish.

Nutrition:
- Calories: 209
- Fat: 8.2g
- Fiber: 6.5g
- Carbs: 35.4 g
- Protein: 4.9g
- Cholesterol 0mg
- Sodium: 12mg

# Sweet Potato Mash

Servings: 2    Prep time:10min    Cook time:1h

### INGREDIENTS

¼ cup of olive oil
3 cups of sweet potatoes
Black pepper to the taste

### DIRECTIONS

Arrange the sweet potatoes on a lined baking sheet, bake in the oven at 375F/190C for 1 hour, cool them down, peel, mash them, and put them in a bowl. Add black pepper and the oil, and whisk well. Divide between plates and serve as a side dish.

Nutrition:
- Calories: 482
- Fat: 25.6 g
- Carbs: 62.4g
- Protein: 3.5g
- Cholesterol: 0mg
- Sodium: 20mg

# Bok Choy Mix

Servings: 2    Prep time:10min    Cook time:15min

## INGREDIENTS

2 tbsps of olive oil

3 tbsps of coconut aminos

1-inch ginger, grated

A pinch of red pepper flakes

4 bok choy heads, cut into quarters

2 garlic cloves, minced

1 tbsp of sesame seeds, toasted

## DIRECTIONS

Heat a pan with the olive oil over medium flame. Add coconut aminos, garlic, pepper flakes, ginger, stir, and cook for 3-4 minutes. Add the bok choy and the sesame seeds, toss, cook for 5 minutes more, divide between plates, and serve as a side dish.

Nutrition:
- Calories: 420
- Fat: 2.9g
- Fiber: 18.4g
- Carbs: 44.4 g
- Protein: 26.9g
- Cholesterol: 0mg
- Sodium:1096mg

# Turnip with Orange

Servings: 2    Prep time:10min    Cook time:15min

## INGREDIENTS

1 tsp of lemon juice

Zest of 2 oranges, grated

2 cups of turnips, sliced

3 tbsps of olive oil

1 tsp of rosemary, chopped

Black pepper to the taste

## DIRECTIONS

Heat a pan with the oil over a medium-high flame. Add turnips, stir, and cook for 5 minutes. Add the lemon juice, black pepper, orange zest, and rosemary, stir, cook for 10 minutes more, divide between plates, and serve as a side dish.

Nutrition:
- Calories: 218
- Fat: 21.4 g
- Carbs: 8.7g
- Protein: 1.1g
- Cholesterol: 0mg
- Sodium: 81mg

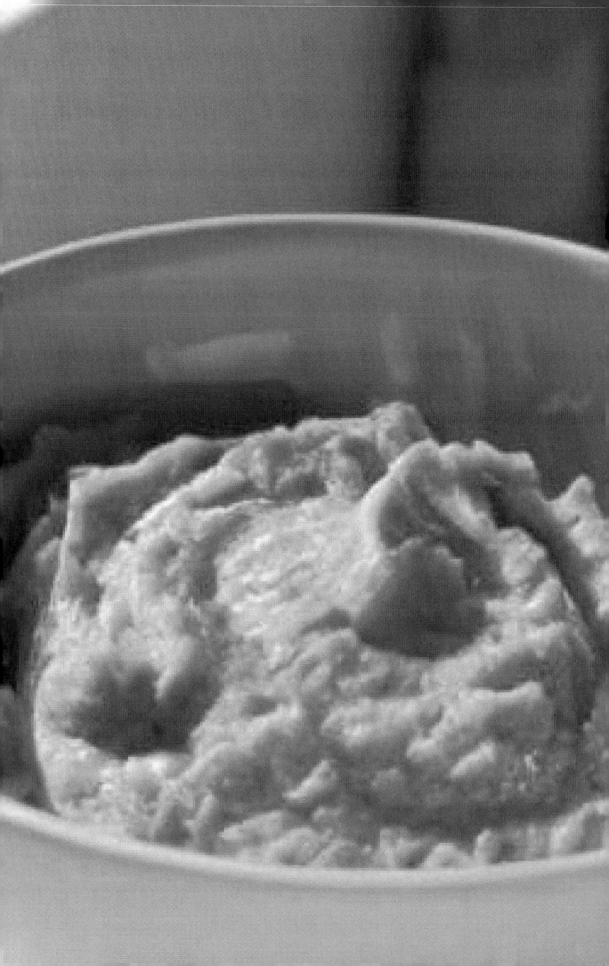

# Fennel Mix

## INGREDIENTS

3 tbsps lemon juice
2 cups fennel, chopped
2 tbsps olive oil
A pinch of black pepper

## DIRECTIONS

Mix fennel with black pepper, oil, and lemon juice in a salad bowl, toss well, divide between plates, and serve as a side dish.

Nutrition:
- Calories: 153
- Fat: 14.4g
- Fiber: 2.8g
- Carbs: 6.9g
- Protein: 1.3g
- Cholesterol: 0mg
- Sodium: 50mg

# Cauliflower Mix

Servings: 2          Prep time:10min          Cook time:35min

## INGREDIENTS

6 cups of cauliflower florets
2 tbsps of sweet paprika
2 cups of chicken stock
¼ cup of avocado oil
Black pepper to the taste

## DIRECTIONS

In a baking dish, combine the cauliflower with stock, oil, black pepper, and paprika, and toss. Bake in the oven at 375F/190C for 35 minutes. Divide between plates and serve as a side dish.

Nutrition:
- Calories: 142
- Fat: 5.3 g
- Carbs: 22.1g
- Protein: 8g
- Cholesterol: 0mg
- Sodium: 857mg

# Spinach and Tomato

Servings: 2    Prep time:20min                Cook time:25min

## INGREDIENTS

1 1/2 cup baby leaf spinach

3 tbsps light soft cheese

2 courgette

1 cup chopped tomatoes

2 cloves garlic, finelly chopped

2 level tbsps freshly grated Parmesan cheese

## DIRECTIONS

Cook the spinach in a saucepan of boiling water over high heat for 1 minute. Drain well and cool slightly. Squeeze the water from the spinach as much as possible. Put it in a food processor with the soft cheese and process until smooth. Season to taste. Preheat the oven to 400F/200C. Peel courgette lengthways into long thin ribbons using a vegetable peeler. Arrange the best 12 ribbons in a single layer on a clean work surface, butting up side by side. Pat dry with kitchen paper and season. Spread the spinach mixture over the courgette strips to cover and roll each strip into a spiral (like Swiss rolls). Over high heat, fry in a pan; roughly chop what is left of your courgettes and garlic and fry for 2-3 minutes or until softened. Remove from the heat, stir in the chopped tomatoes, and season. Spoon the tomatoes into an oven-proof dish and spread it out to cover the base. Arrange the courgette spirals on their sides in the tomato sauce, sprinkle with the Parmesan, and bake for 20 minutes or until bubbling. Serve hot.

Nutrition:
- Calories: 243
- Fat: 11.8g
- Fiber: 4.5g
- Carbs: 16.9g
- Protein: 18.1g
- Cholesterol: 20mg
- Sodium: 405mg

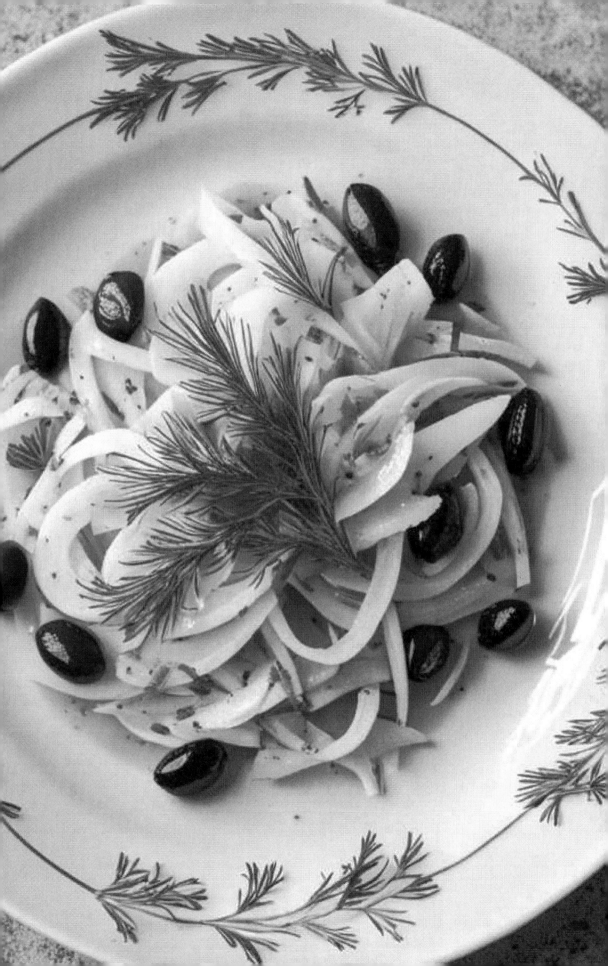

# Popquorn

Servings: 2      Prep time:10min                  Cook time:30min

## INGREDIENTS

2 tbsp Cajun seasoning

2 eggs, beaten

2 tbsps cornflakes crushed

3/4 cup Quorn Chicken style pieces

1 little gem lettuce

Nutrition:
- Calories: 366
- Fat: 15.2g
- Fiber: 6.6g
- Carbs: 31.2g
- Protein: 19.2g
- Cholesterol: 164mg
- Sodium: 1075mg

## DIRECTIONS

Preheat oven to 400F/200C. Put the Cajun seasoning in a shallow bowl, the beaten eggs in a second shallow bowl, and the crushed cornflakes in a third. Pat the Quorn pieces dry with kitchen paper and toss in the Cajun seasoning. Dip the seasoned Quorn in the eggs and the cornflakes to coat well. Arrange the Quorn on a baking tray and bake for 20 - 25 minutes or until crisp. Separate the Little Gem leaves, arrange the largest leaves on plates, and top with the popquorn to serve.

# Lentil and Kale Ragu

Servings: 2      Prep time:10min                  Cook time:40min

## INGREDIENTS

1 cup mixed casserole veg

1 cup passata

2 tbsp soy sauce

1 cup green lentil from can, drained and rinsed

2 tbsps kale roughly chopped

Nutrition:
- Calories: 238
- Fat: 0.8 g
- Carbs: 42.4g
- Protein: 14.7g
- Cholesterol: 0mg
- Sodium: 913mg

## DIRECTIONS

Add the casserole veg in a pan over medium heat, cover, and cook for 8-10 minutes, occasionally stirring ad water if necessary.

Add the passata and soy sauce and season with black pepper. Pour 200 ml water into the passata container, shake well, and add to the pan. Bring to a boil over high heat, then cover, reduce the heat to low, and simmer for 20 minutes. Stir in the lentils and kale and simmer for 5 minutes. Season to taste and serve hot.

# Aubergine Skewers

Servings: 2    Prep time: 10min         Cook time: 25min

## INGREDIENTS

1 cucumber

2 tbsp rice vinegar seasoned

2 tbsp soy sauce

1 medium aubergine thinly sliced lengthways

8 spring onions, each cut into 3 pieces

Nutrition:
- Calories: 59
- Fat: 0.3g
- Fiber: 3.6g
- Carbs: 12.3g
- Protein: 3.1g
- Cholesterol 0mg
- Sodium 915mg

## DIRECTIONS

Using a vegetable peeler, peel the cucumber into ribbons and place it in a large bowl. Pour over 2 tsp vinegar and mix well, then cover and chill. Mix the remaining vinegar with the soy sauce and set aside. Steam the aubergine slices for 5 minutes to soften. Cool slightly. Fold the aubergine slices and thread them on 4 skewers with the spring onions. Brush with a little soy mixture, and season with black pepper. Place a large nonstick griddle pan over high heat. Grill the skewers for 8-10 minutes, turning frequently and basting with the remaining marinade from time to time until charred, soft, and smoky.

# Jacket Potato

Servings: 2         Prep time: 15min         Cook time: 50min

## INGREDIENTS

2 large sweet potatoes

4 spring onion

1 cup baked beans in tomato sauce

1/2 cup cherry tomatoes halved

1 tbsp feta cheese crumbled

Nutrition:
- Calories 303
- Fat: 5.9 g
- Carbs: 54.8g
- Protein: 12.5g
- Cholesterol 22mg
- Sodium 792 mg

## DIRECTIONS

Preheat the oven to 400F/200C. Scrub the sweet potatoes, prick them with a fork, and arrange them on a nonstick baking tray. Bake for 45 minutes or until tender. Shred the green parts of the spring onions and put them in a bowl of cold water. Cover and set aside until ready to use. Thinly slice the white parts of the spring onions and put them in a small saucepan with the baked beans and cherry tomatoes. Heat until the tomatoes have softened. Halve the sweet potatoes, divide them between plates, and spoon over the bean mixture. Scatter over the shredded spring onions and the feta, season to taste, and serve hot.

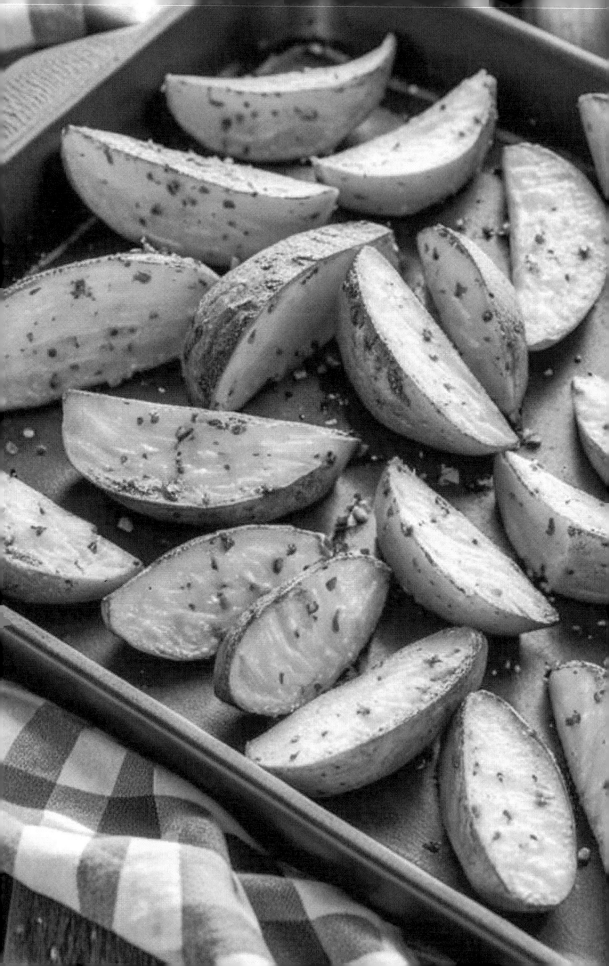

# Roasted Cauliflower

Servings: 2    Prep time: 15min            Cook time: 40min

## INGREDIENTS

1 small cauliflower – 2 cups
1 red onion cut into thin wedges
½ garlic bulb halved through
the cloves
1 lemon grated zest and juice
1 tsp za'atar spice

Nutrition:
- Calories: 56
- Fat: 0.2g
- Fiber: 4.5g
- Carbs: 12.4g
- Protein: 3.3g
- Cholesterol 0mg
- Sodium 42mg

## DIRECTIONS

Preheat the oven to 400F/200C. Break the cauliflower into florets and boil over high heat for 2 – 3 minutes. Drain well and spread out in a single layer in a large roasting tin lined with nonstick baking paper. Add the onion wedges and garlic bulb to the tin and sprinkle over the lemon zest, juice, and za'atar spice. Toss well and roast for 20-30 minutes or until the cauliflower is tender and beginning to turn golden brown. Squeeze the garlic flesh from the bulbs, mash in a bowl, and toss through the cauliflower. Serve hot with lemon wedges to squeeze over.

# Beetroot Burgers

Servings: 2    Prep time: 10min            Cook time: 45min

## INGREDIENTS

3 large sweet potatoes
peeled
2 large parsnips peeled
1 level tbsp plain flour
small pack of fresh mint
finely chopped
1 cup g beetroot peeled
and coarsely grated

Nutrition:
- Calories 243
- Fat: 0.1g
- Carbs: 54.7g
- Protein: 6.6g
- Cholesterol 0mg
- Sodium 160mg

## DIRECTIONS

Preheat oven to 400F/200C. Finely chop 1 sweet potato and cook in a saucepan of boiling water for 8 minutes or until tender. Drain and return to the pan for 30-40 seconds to remove excess moisture. Remove from the heat and mash, then tip into a bowl and stir in the flour and mint. Squeeze out any excess liquid from the grated beetroot. Add to the sweet potato mixture and mix well. Season, shape into burgers, and arrange on a baking tray. Cut the remaining sweet potatoes and the parsnips, and spread them out in a single layer on a large baking tray. Season lightly and bake on the top shelf of the oven for 30 minutes. Put the burger tray in the middle of the oven and bake for 20 minutes. Serve hot.

# Roasted Potatoes Wedges

Servings: 2     Prep time:10min          Cook time:55min

## INGREDIENTS

2 big potatoes
2 tbsps olive oil
1/2 cup grated cheese
salt
pepper
2 garlic cloves, finely chooped
1 small red onion chopped

## DIRECTIONS

Preheat oven to 350F/180C. Cut each potato lengthwise in half. Cut each half into 3 wedges. In a large bowl, sprinkle potatoes with oil and all other ingredients. Toss to coat. Arrange potatoes in a single layer on a baking pan coated with cooking paper. Sprinkle with any remaining coating. Bake until golden brown and tender, 45-55 minutes.

Nutrition:
- Calories: 510
- Fat: 23.8g
- Fiber: 9.4g
- Carbs: 63.4g
- Protein: 13.7g
- Cholesterol 30mg
- Sodium 277mg

# Broccoli in Oven

Servings: 2     Prep time:15min          Cook time:40min

## INGREDIENTS

2 small broccoli crowns
3 tbsp olive oil
salt pepper
1 tbsp crushed rep pepper flakes
4 garlic cloves thinly sliced
2 tbsp grated cheese
1 tbsp grated lemon zest
2 tbsp of sunflower seeds

## DIRECTIONS

Preheat oven to 400F/200C. Cut broccoli crowns into quarters from top to bottom. Drizzle with oil and sprinkle with salt, pepper, and pepper flakes. Place in a parchment-lined pan. Roast for 10-12 minutes. Sprinkle with garlic, and roast for 2 minutes. Sprinkle with cheese and roast until cheese is melted and stalks of broccoli are tender. Sprinkle with lemon zest and seeds.

Nutrition:
- Calories 263
- Fat: 25g
- Carbs: 8.3g
- Protein: 5.7g
- Cholesterol 7mg
- Sodium 137mg

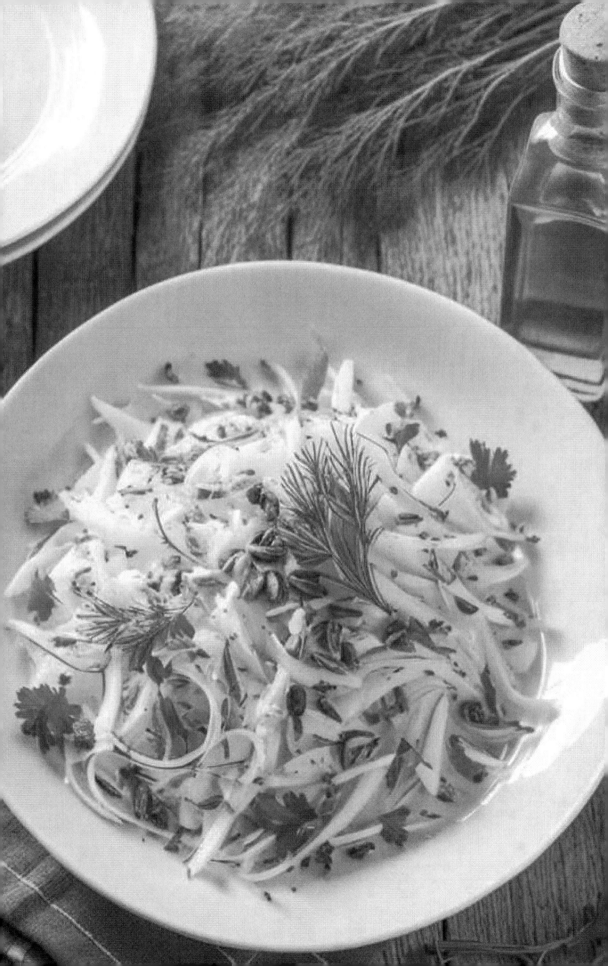

# SIDES

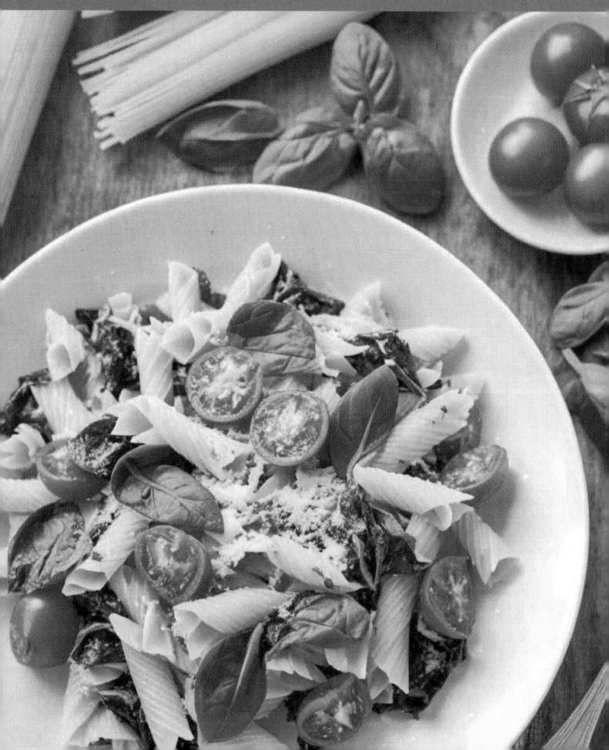

# Couscous Simple

INGREDIENTS

1 cup couscous

2 cups water

salt

1 tbsp olive oil

2 tbsp soya sauce

DIRECTIONS

Fry couscous in a pan with olive oil and stir with a wooden spoon until it changes color; put it in a bowl through over salted boiling water and soya sauce and cover. Wait for around 15 min so the couscous will absorb all water and double the volume. Serve as a side dish.

Nutrition:
- Calories: 394
- Fat: 7.6g
- Fiber: 4.5g
- Carbs: 68.2
- Protein: 12g
- Cholesterol 0mg
- Sodium 995mg

# Couscous with Tomatoes

Servings: 2          Prep time:15min          Cook time:15min

INGREDIENTS

1 cup couscous

1 1/2 cup water

4 tomatoes

1 bunch of parsley

1 tsp cumin seeds

1 bunch leaf of mint

1 bunch leaf of basil

2 springs onion

1 tbsp olive oil

salt

DIRECTIONS

Fry couscous in a pan with olive oil stir all the time with wooden spon until it changes the color. Put the couscous in the bowl through over salted boiling water nad cover. Leave for 15 min.

Put the couscous on a serving plate. Wash, dry and cut the tomatoes in slices and put on couscous, chop parsley, mint, basil and spring onion and mix in the couscous.

Nutrition:
- Calories 451
- Fat: 8.7g
- Carbs: 79.7g
- Protein: 15.2g
- Cholesterol 0mg
- Sodium 123mg

# Couscous with Vegetables

Servings: 2      Prep time:10min              Cook time:20min

## INGREDIENTS

1 cup couscous

2 cups water

2 onions

3 carrots

2 courgettes

2 garlic cloves

rosemary

1 bunch mint

2 tbsp olive oil

salt

Nutrition:
- Calories: 567
- Fat: 2.2g
- Fiber: 11.8g
- Carbs: 94.7g
- Protein: 15.8g
- Cholesterol 0mg
- Sodium 183mg

## DIRECTIONS

Boil water with mint and salt. Put the couscous in the bowl through boiling water with mint and cover. Leave for 15 min. Wash and cut long-way carrots and courgettes. Cut the onion and fry them in a pan with oil until soft. Add garlic and fry for 1 min more. Add carrots, and after 5 min, add courgettes. Finally, add finely cut rosemary and salt, cover the pan, and let on medium heat for 10 min. Stir couscous with vegetables and serve.

# Basil Pasta

Servings: 2          Prep time:15min+2h    Cook time:10min

## INGREDIENTS

1 cup of pasta

1 bunch of fresh basil

2 cloves of garlic

1/2 cup  green olives

2 tbsps of grated Parmesan cheese

olive oil

salt

Nutrition:
- Calories 363
- Fat: 15.8g
- Carbs: 45.1g
- Protein: 13.4g
- Cholesterol 20mg
- Sodium 563mg

## DIRECTIONS

Finely chop garlic, basil, and olives. Then put everything to macerate in oil for about a couple of hours. Boil the pasta in plenty of salted water, drain, and pour into the bowl where you have macerated the sauce; add the grated Parmesan cheese and a little oil, mix well, and serve.

# Pasta with Walnuts

## INGREDIENTS

1 cup of noodles
1/4 cup of cooking cream
a handful of walnuts
2 tbsps of fresh cheese
salt

## DIRECTIONS

Boil the noodles in a pot with plenty of salted water, as per instructions on the package. Melt the chopped cheese with the cream over low heat in a saucepan. Mix until well blended, and add the cut walnut kernels. Mix pasta and sauce when everything is still hot and serve.

Nutrition:
- Calories: 369
- Fat: 26.5g
- Fiber: 3g
- Carbs: 25.3g
- Protein: 11.2g
- Cholesterol 31mg
- Sodium 150mg

# Pasta and Walnuts 2

## INGREDIENTS

1 cup g of spaghetti
1/2 cup of walnut kernels
bunch of basil
2 tbsp of grated Parmesan cheese
1/2 cup of ripe cherry tomatoes,
olive oil,
salt and pepper

## DIRECTIONS

Coarsely chop the walnut kernels and toast everything in a non-stick pan. Combine the walnuts, the chopped basil, the cheese, a little salt, ground pepper, and 4 tbsp of oil in the blender until creamy pesto. Cut the cherry tomatoes into wedges. Mix the spaghetti boiled al dente with the pesto, add the cherry tomatoes, mix, and serve.

Nutrition:
- Calories 882
- Fat: 44.8g
- Carbs: 94g
- Protein: 31.9g
- Cholesterol 20mg
- Sodium 269mg

# Pasta with Beans

Servings: 2    Prep time:15min         Cook time:20min

## INGREDIENTS

1/2 cup frozen peas

1/4 cup frozen broad beans

1 tbsp olive oil

1 small leek, finely sliced

1 tsp dried chilli flakes

3 tbsp ricotta

1 tbs parmesan grated, plus a little extra to serve

1/2 lemon, zested and juiced

1 cup linguine

a small bunch mint

Nutrition:
- Calories: 618
- Fat: 18.1g
- Fiber: 4g
- Carbs: 86.7g
- Protein: 29.23g
- Cholesterol 121mg
- Sodium 360mg

## DIRECTIONS

Put the peas and broad beans into a bowl and pour over a kettle of boiling water. Leave for 1 minute, and drain. Blend them in a food processor with 1 tbsp of water until smooth. Heat the olive oil in a frying pan and fry the leek with seasoning for 8-10 minutes until soft. Stir in the chili flakes, broad beans, and peas puree and fry for 2 minutes. Cool slightly and put into a bowl with the ricotta, parmesan, lemon zest, and juice, and mix well. Cook the linguine following pack instructions, reserving some cooking water. Tip the pasta back into the pan, add the pea and leek mix, and a splash of the cooking water. Mix well and serve with the mint and more parmesan.

# Pasta with Broccoli

Servings: 2    Prep time:20min         Cook time:20min

## INGREDIENTS

1 cup bellaverde broccoli

1 cup tagliatelle

1/2 cup skinless and boneless salmon fillets

1/2 cup dry white wine

1 tbsp butter

4 spring onions, finely sliced

1 cup single cream

Chopped fresh dill to garnish, if liked

Salt and freshly ground black pepper

Nutrition:
- Calories 675
- Fat: 26.4g
- Carbs: 93.2g
- Protein: 13.5g
- Cholesterol 76mg
- Sodium 245mg

## DIRECTIONS

Boil the tagliatelle as per package instructions. Drain well. While the pasta cooks, place the salmon in a medium frying pan and add the white wine, salt, and pepper. Cover, boil, then simmer for 5-6 mins or until the salmon is cooked and flakes easily. Transfer the salmon to a plate and break it into large bits with a fork. Increase the heat and simmer the cooking liquid until reduced to about 45ml (3tbsps).
Meanwhile, wash and prepare the broccoli by trimming the base of each spear and chopping the remaining into 3cm/1.5-inch pieces. Add the butter to the reduced wine, then add the spring onions, broccoli, and sauté for 3 mins. Add the cream, cover, and simmer for 3-4 mins or until the broccoli is tender. Remove the lid, stir in the salmon, add the sauce to the cooked tagliatelle, then toss until coated in the sauce. Serve sprinkled with a bit of dill.

# Spagetti with Aubergine

Servings: 2     Prep time:10min+marin.     Cook time:35min

## INGREDIENTS

1 cup spagetti
2 Aubergines medium the
long one
2 cloves of garlic
1 bunch of parsley
olive oil
salt

Nutrition:
- Calories: 513
- Fat: 1g
- Fiber: 13.5g
- Carbs: 87.3g
- Protein: 15.1g
- Cholesterol 0mg
- Sodium 95mg

## DIRECTIONS

Wash and dry the aubergines, cut them into slices, and salt them. In this way, the water will drain. After a couple of hours, drain them well and fry them in a pan with plenty of oil, to which you have also added garlic. Drain oil with a kitchen roll. Boil the pasta as per instructions on the box, drain well, and mix with aubergines in a salad bowl with chopped parsley. Serve hot.

# Simple Rice

Servings: 2     Prep time:15min     Cook time:30min

## INGREDIENTS

1 tbsp olive oil
1 cup long-grain white rice
2 cloves of garlic
2 cups low-sodium chicken broth
1 pinch salt, or to taste

Nutrition:
- Calories 149
- Fat: 3 g
- Carbs: 27g
- Protein: 4g
- Cholesterol 1mg
- Sodium 94 mg

## DIRECTIONS

Heat olive oil in a non-stick saucepan over medium-high with finely chopped garlic for 1 min. Add the rice and stir in the hot oil quickly to toast the rice, 3 to 4 minutes. Pour chicken broth over the rice mixture, season with salt, and bring to a boil; reduce heat to low, place a cover on the saucepan, and cook until the broth is absorbed and the rice is tender, about 20 minutes. Remove from heat and rest for 5 minutes before lifting the lid.

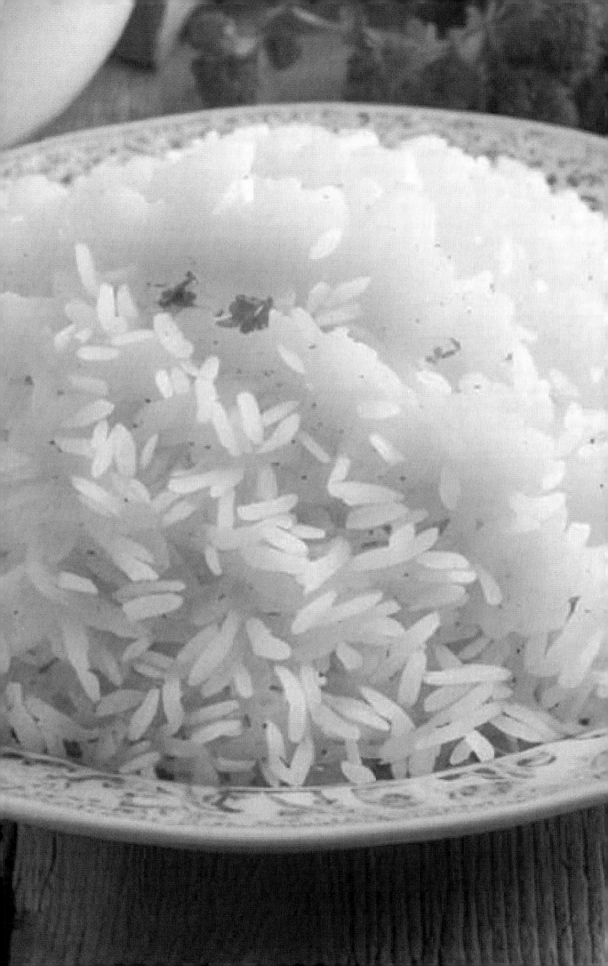

# Orzo Pasta and Rice

Servings: 2    Prep time:10min                    Cook time:25min

## INGREDIENTS

2 tbsp olive oil

1/4 cup orzo pasta

1/4 cup long-grain rice

2 cups chicken or
vegetables broth

salt

## DIRECTIONS

Heat olive oil over medium heat in a large, heavy saucepan; add orzo and brown until golden. Add rice and broth; boil, cover, and lower heat to medium-low. Simmer for about 20 to 25 minutes or until all water is absorbed. Serve as a side dish.

Nutrition:
- Calories: 192
- Fat: 5g
- Fiber: 1g
- Carbs: 32 g
- Protein: 5g
- Cholesterol 12mg
- Sodium 265mg

# Creamy Orzo Pasta

Servings: 2         Prep time:15min                    Cook time:15min

## INGREDIENTS

2 tbsp olive oil
2 tbsp butter
1 small onion finely chopped
2 cloves garlic finely chopped
1/4 cup Sliced baby Bella mushrooms
1/2 cup Dry Orzo pasta
2 cups Chicken broth
Freshly grated Parmesan cheese
salt and pepper

Nutrition:
- Calories: 471
- Fat: 23g
- Carbs: 46g
- Protein: 20g
- Cholesterol 68mg
- Sodium 422mg

## DIRECTIONS

Heat 2 tbsp olive oil in a skillet over medium-high heat. Then add onions and mushrooms and fry until the mushrooms are tender. Season with salt and pepper. Add garlic and fry for 1 minute more. Remove and set aside. In the same skillet, add the butter, melt, and add the orzo, stirring for about 1 minute or 2. Do not let it burn. Pour in chicken broth. Bring to a boil - reduce heat to medium/low and cover and let it cook for about 5 -6 minutes or until the orzo is tender. Return the mushrooms mixture to the skillet, together with the parmesan cheese. Mix thoroughly to incorporate mushrooms and cheese. Add spinach. Mix well - remove from heat. Adjust seasonings to taste. Serve immediately.

# Tomato Pasta

INGREDIENTS

1 cup ripe tomatoes, halved

2 cloves garlic, skin on

2 tbsp extra-virgin olive oil

1/2 tsp black pepper

2 cups  spaghetti

a handful of leaves basil

DIRECTIONS

In a pot over medium heat, fry the garlic in olive oil. Add halved tomatoes and pepper. Let it sim for 15 min. In the meantime, boil spaghetti in water as per instructions on the package. Drain the pasta, stir it in tomato source in the pan, and let it cook for a 1-minute string to coat. Serve on a plate and spring with basil leaves.

Nutrition:
- Calories: 511
- Fat: 17.2g
- Fiber: 1.3g
- Carbs: 74.9g
- Protein: 15.5g
- Cholesterol 93mg
- Sodium 38mg

# Rice in Oven

INGREDIENTS

2 tbsp. olive oil

1 lemon

1 small onion, chopped

1 cloves garlic, chopped

1/2 cup rice

2 cups vegetable broth

salt

1/2 cup grated Parmesan

1 cup peas,

ground black pepper

Chopped fresh parsley, for garnish

Nutrition:
- Calories 647
- Fat: 31.3 g
- Carbs: 59.3g
- Protein: 36.3g
- Cholesterol 50mg
- Sodium 1516mg

DIRECTIONS

Preheat oven to 375F/190C. Melt 2 tbsp of butter in a pot (you can use it in the oven) over medium-high heat. Add onion and lemon zest to the olive oil and cook, often stirring, until softened, about 5 minutes. Add garlic and cook, stirring, until fragrant, about 1 minute. Stir in rice, broth, and salt. Bring to a simmer, cover, and transfer to the oven. Bake until rice is tender, 20 minutes. Carefully remove the lid and stir in Parmesan, peas, and pepper until the peas are warm. Cut the lemon in half and squeeze half the juice into the risotto; stir to combine. Remove the lemon zest and serve topped with parsley.

# Corn Grit with Cheeses

Servings: 2    Prep time:10min    Cook time:10min

## INGREDIENTS

1 cup low-sodium chicken broth
1 cup water
salt
1/2 cup corn grits
2 tbsp butter, divided
1/2 cup shredded cheddar
1/4 cup grated Parmesan
black pepper

Nutrition:
- Calories: 341
- Fat: 23.3g
- Fiber: 0.2g
- Carbs: 10.3g
- Protein: 23.8g
- Cholesterol 66mg
- Sodium 1242mg

## DIRECTIONS

Bring broth and water to a boil in a medium saucepan and season generously with salt. Reduce heat and then whisk in grits. Simmer, often stirring, until grits have absorbed the liquid and are tender for 10 minutes. Remove from heat.
Stir in butter and cheese and season with pepper.

# Coconut Rice

Servings: 2    Prep time:20min    Cook time:20min

## INGREDIENTS

1 cup long grain rice
1/2 cup coconut milk
3/4 cup water
salt
Toasted sesame seeds, for garnish (optional)

Nutrition:
- Calories 527
- Fat: 19.4g
- Carbs: 79.4g
- Protein: 9.6g
- Cholesterol 0mg
- Sodium 95mg

## DIRECTIONS

Combine rice, coconut milk, water, and salt in a large pot over medium heat. Bring to a boil, then reduce heat, and let simmer, covered, for 18 to 20 minutes or until rice is tender. Remove from heat and let sit for 10 minutes, then fluff with a fork. Serve topped with sesame seeds.

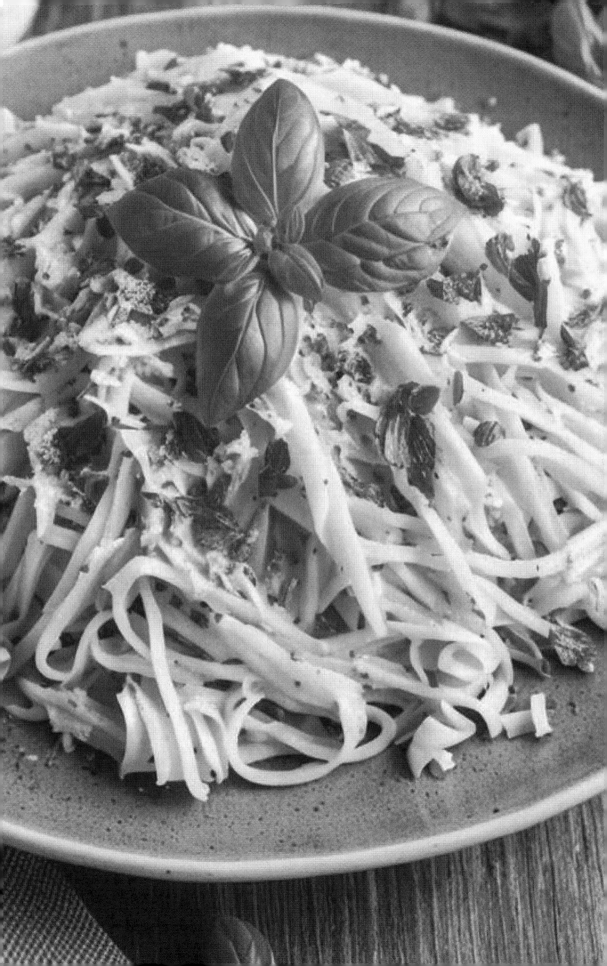

# Orzo with Basil

Servings: 2    Prep time:5min                    Cook time:18min

## INGREDIENTS

1/2 cup orzo pasta
2 tbsp butter
1/2 cup chicken broth
1/4 cup grated cheese
2 tsps dried basil
pepper
Thinly sliced fresh basil

## DIRECTIONS

In a large skillet, saute orzo in butter until lightly browned, 3-5 minutes. Stir in broth. Bring to a boil. Reduce heat; cover and simmer until liquid is absorbed and orzo is tender, 10-15 minutes. Stir in the cheese, basil, and pepper. Top with fresh basil.

Nutrition:
- Calories: 285
- Fat: 10g
- Fiber: 1g
- Carbs: 38 g
- Protein: 11g
- Cholesterol 26mg
- Sodium 641mg

# Noodles and Basil

Servings: 2        Prep time:10min                Cook time:10min

## INGREDIENTS

1 cup wide egg noodles
2 tbsp shredded cheese
1 tbsp butter
1 tbsp olive oil
2 tbsp minced fresh basil
1/2 tbsp minced fresh thyme
1 garlic clove, minced
salt

## DIRECTIONS

In a large saucepan, boil noodles according to package directions; drain. Add the remaining ingredients and toss to coat.

Nutrition:
- Calories 243
- Fat: 15 g
- Carbs: 21g
- Protein: 6g
- Cholesterol 46mg
- Sodium 444 mg

# Creamy Pasta

Servings: 2    Prep time:10min        Cook time:10min

INGREDIENTS
1 cup bow-tie pasta
1 tbsp butter
1 tbsp olive oil
1 tbsp all-purpose flour
1/2 tbsp minced garlic
salt
dried basil
crushed red pepper flakes
1 tbsp milk
1 tbsp chicken broth
1 tbsp water
2 tbsp shredded cheese
1 tbsp sour cream

Nutrition:
- Calories: 196
- Fat: 12g
- Fiber: 1g
- Carbs: 17 g
- Protein: 6g
- Cholesterol 19mg
- Sodium 252mg

DIRECTIONS
Cook pasta according to package directions. In a small saucepan, melt butter. Stir in the oil, flour, garlic, and seasonings until blended. Gradually add the milk, broth, and water. Bring to a boil; cook and stir until slightly thickened, about 2 minutes. Remove from the heat; stir in cheese and sour cream. Drain pasta; toss with sauce.

# Quinoa with Bacon

Servings: 2    Prep time:15min        Cook time:40min

INGREDIENTS
1/4 cup almonds
1 tsp vegetable oil
2 thick slices bacon,
cut into 1/4-inch dice
1 small shallot, minced
1 cup quinoa, rinsed
2 cups chicken broth
1 sage sprig
1 tsp minced chives
1 tsp chopped parsley
Salt and ground pepper

Nutrition:
- Calories 553
- Fat: 22.8g
- Carbs: 60.4g
- Protein: 26.8g
- Cholesterol 21mg
- Sodium 1208mg

DIRECTIONS
In a medium saucepan, heat the oil. Add the bacon and cook over high heat until the fat has rendered, about 2 minutes. Add the shallot and fry, stirring until softened but not browned, about 1 minute. Add the quinoa, broth, sage, salt, and pepper, and boil. Cover and cook on low heat until the stock has been absorbed, about 17 minutes. Remove the quinoa from the heat and let stand, covered, for 5 minutes. Discard the sage and fluff the quinoa with a fork. Stir in the chives, parsley, and toasted almonds, and serve.

149

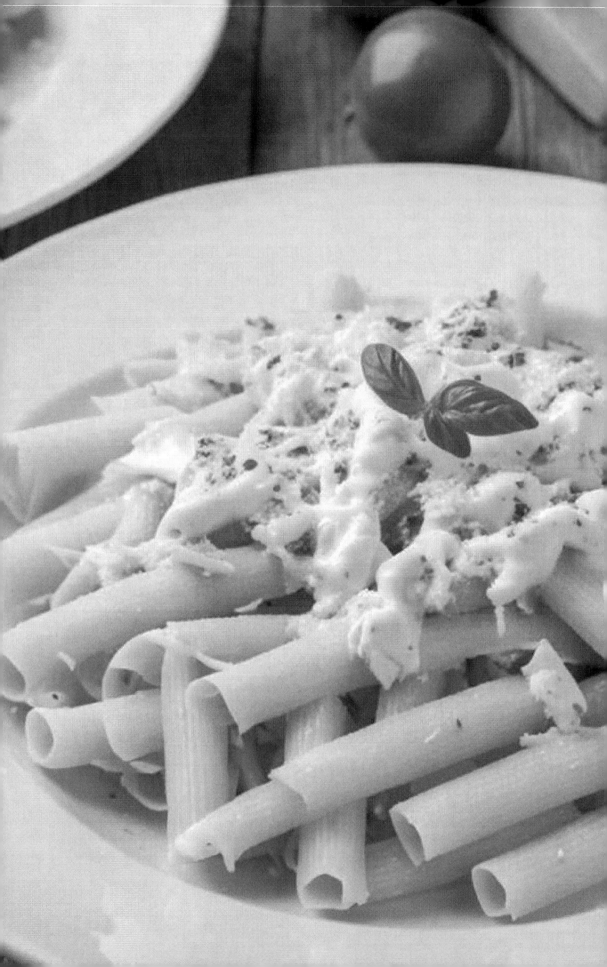

# DESSERTS

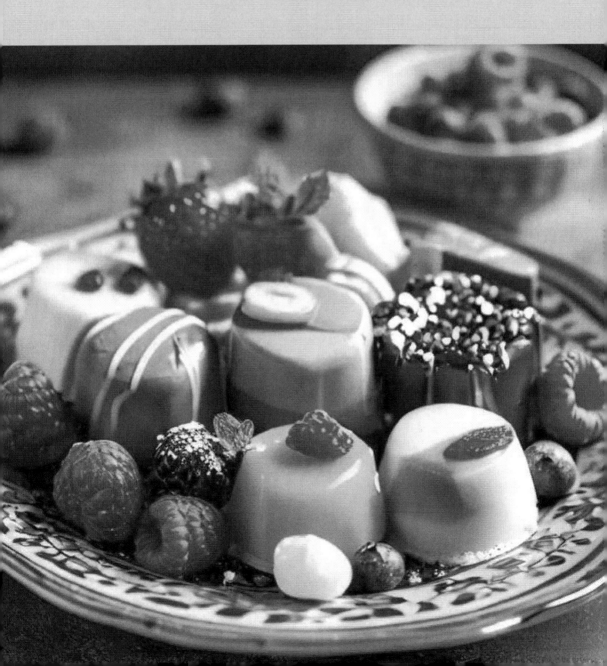

# Pancake

## INGREDIENTS

½ cup of almond flour

2 scoops of Stevia

½ tsp of cinnamon

2 eggs

1/2 cup of cream cheese

## DIRECTIONS

Put all the ingredients in a blender and blend until smooth. Dish out the mixture to a medium bowl and set aside. Heat the butter in a skillet over medium fire and add one-quarter of the mix. Spread the mixture and cook for about 4 minutes on both sides until golden brown. Repeat with the rest of the mixture in batches and serve warm.

Nutrition:
- Calories: 309
- Fat: 27.9g
- Fiber: 1.1g
- Carbs: 3.9g
- Protein: 11.4g
- Cholesterol 227mg
- Sodium 236mg

# Cocoa Drink

Servings: 2        Prep time:15min              Cook time:0min

## INGREDIENTS

2 cups of cream, whipped

1 tsp of cocoa powder

1 tsp of peanut butter

½ cup of coconut milk

2 tbsp of Stevia

½ tsp of vanilla extract

## DIRECTIONS

Mix up the coconut milk and whipped cream. Add the cocoa powder and mix it with the help of the hand mixer. Add peanut butter, vanilla extract, and Stevia when the liquid is homogenous. Whisk it well. Pour into the serving glasses.

Nutrition:
- Calories 313
- Fat: 29.1g
- Carbs: 12g
- Protein: 4.1g
- Cholesterol 46mg
- Sodium 100mg

# Marshmallows

Servings: 2    Prep time:10min                Cook time:0min

## INGREDIENTS

12 scoops of stevia

2 tbsps of gelatin

¾ cup of sugar

1/2 cup of cold water

2 tsps of vanilla extract

1/2 cup of hot water

## DIRECTIONS

Mix the gelatin with cold water; stir and leave aside for 5 minutes. Put hot water in a pan, add sugar and stevia, and stir well. Combine this with the gelatin mix, add vanilla extract, beat it using a mixer, and pour it into a baking pan. Leave aside in the fridge until it sets, then cut into pieces and serve.

Nutrition:
- Calories: 317
- Fat: 0g
- Fiber: 0g
- Carbs: 75.5g
- Protein: 6g
- Cholesterol 0mg
- Sodium 16mg

# Mug Cake

Servings: 2        Prep time:5min            Cook time:10min

## INGREDIENTS

4 tbsps of almond meal

1 tbsp of coconut flour

2 tbsps of ghee

1 tbsp of stevia

1/4 tsp of vanilla extract

1/2 tsp of baking powder

1 tbsp of cocoa powder

1 egg

## DIRECTIONS

Put the ghee in a mug and introduce it in the microwave for a few seconds. Add cocoa powder, stevia, egg, baking powder, vanilla, and coconut flour and stir well. Add almond meal as well; stir again, introduce in the microwave, and cook for 2 minutes. Serve your mug cake with blueberries on top.

Nutrition:
- Calories 251
- Fat: 22.2 g
- Carbs: 8.9g
- Protein: 6.8g
- Cholesterol 115mg
- Sodium 48mg

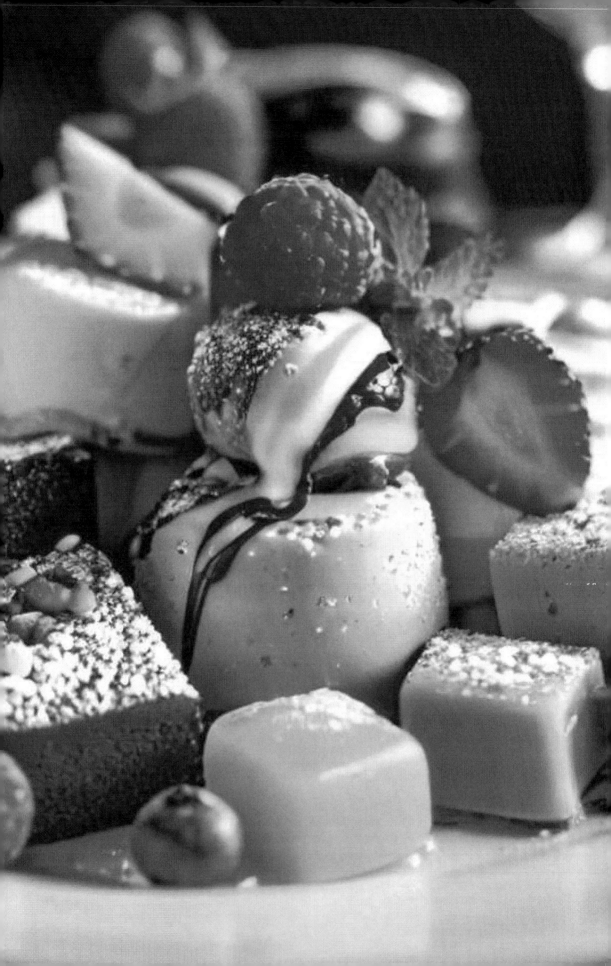

# Orange Cake

Servings: 2    Prep time:30min          Cook time:20min

## INGREDIENTS

1 orange; cut into quarters

1 tsp of vanilla extract

1 tsp of baking powder

1/2 cup of cream cheese

1/2 cup of coconut yogurt

2 cups of almond meal

2 tbsps of orange zest

2 tbsps of stevia

6 eggs

A pinch of salt

Nutrition:
- Calories: 1026
- Fat: 83.5g
- Fiber: 14.2g
- Carbs: 37.3g
- Protein: 42.7g
- Cholesterol 555mg
- Sodium 448mg

## DIRECTIONS

In your food processor, pulse the orange very well. Add the almond meal, eggs, baking powder, vanilla extract, and a pinch of salt, and beat well again. Transfer this into 2 springform pans, introduce in the oven at 350F/176C, and bake for 20 minutes. Meanwhile, in a bowl, mix the cream cheese with orange zest, coconut yogurt, and stevia, and stir well. Place one cake layer on a plate, add half of the cream cheese mix, add the other cake layer, and top with the rest of the cream cheese mix. Spread it well, slice, and serve.

# Pumpkin Custard

Servings: 2    Prep time:15min          Cook time:40min

## INGREDIENTS

2 cups of coconut milk

2 cups of pumpkin puree

2 tsps of vanilla extract

8 scoops of stevia

3 tbsps of Erythritol

1 tsp of gelatin

1/4 cup of warm water

A pinch of salt

1 tsp of cinnamon powder

## DIRECTIONS

Mix pumpkin puree with coconut milk, a pinch of salt, vanilla extract, cinnamon powder, stevia, and Erythritol; stir well and heat up for a few minutes. In a bowl, mix gelatin and water and stir. Combine the 2 mixtures; stir well, divide custard into ramekins, and leave aside to cool down. Keep in the fridge until served.

Nutrition:
- Calories 659
- Fat: 57.9g
- Carbs: 41.2g
- Protein: 11.2g
- Cholesterol 0mg
- Sodium 134mg

# Chocolate Truffles

Servings: 2    Prep time: 15min          Cook time: 10min

## INGREDIENTS

1 cup of chocolate chips
2 tbsps of butter
2 tsps of brandy
2 tbsps of sugar
2/3 cup of heavy cream
1/4 tsp of vanilla extract
Cocoa powder

## DIRECTIONS

Put the heavy cream in a heatproof bowl, add butter, sugar, and chocolate chips; stir, introduce in the microwave, and heat up for 1 minute.
Leave it aside for 5 minutes. Then stir well and mix with brandy and vanilla. Stir again, and leave aside in the fridge for a couple of hours. Use a melon baller to shape your truffles, roll them in cocoa powder and serve.

Nutrition:
- Calories: 762
- Fat: 51.9g
- Fiber: 4.5g
- Carbs: 66.1g
- Protein: 8.4g
- Cholesterol 105mg
- Sodium 164mg

# Coconut Pudding

Servings: 2    Prep time: 20min          Cook time: 10min

## INGREDIENTS

1 2/3 cups of coconut milk
1/2 tsp of vanilla extract
3 egg yolks
1 tbsp of gelatin
6 tbsps of Muscovado

## DIRECTIONS

Mix gelatin with 1 tbsp of coconut milk; stir well and leave aside for now. Put the rest of the milk into a pan and heat up over medium fire. Add the Muscovado, stir, and cook for 5 minutes. Mix egg yolks with hot coconut milk and vanilla extract; stir well and return everything to the pan. Cook for 4 minutes. Add gelatin and stir well. Divide this into 2 ramekins and keep it in the fridge until served.

Nutrition:
- Calories 764
- Fat: 54.3g
- Carbs: 54.6g
- Protein: 20.6g
- Cholesterol 315mg
- Sodium 70mg

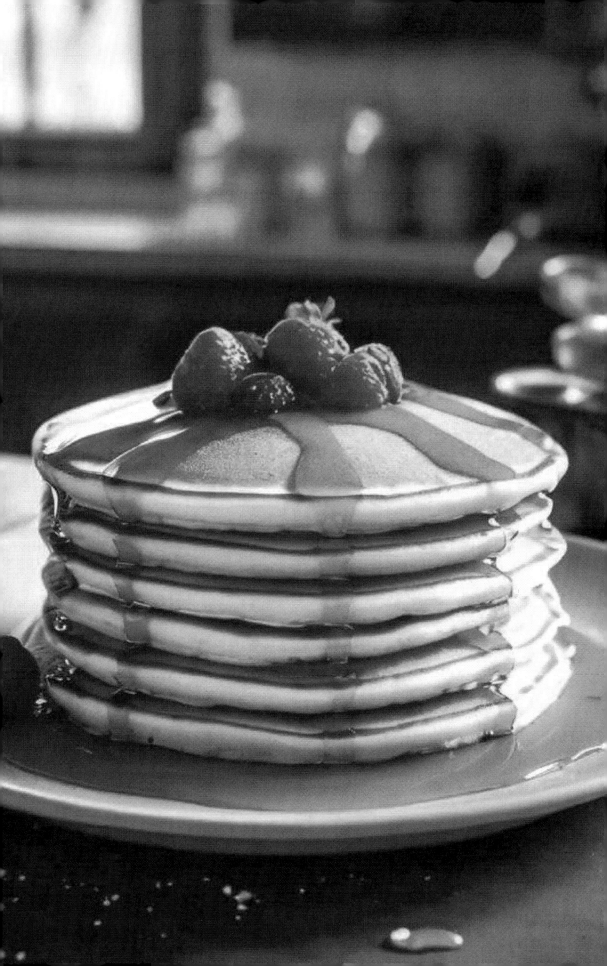

# Easy Macaroons

Servings: 2    Prep time: 20min    Cook time: 10min

## INGREDIENTS

2 cups of coconut; shredded
1 tsp of vanilla extract
4 eggs whites
2 tbsps of stevia
nougat cream

## DIRECTIONS

Mix egg whites with stevia in a bowl and beat using your mixer. Add coconut and vanilla extract and stir. Roll this mixture into small balls and place them on a lined baking sheet. Introduce in the oven at 350F/176C and bake for 10 minutes. Let them cold down. Stick together two pieces with nougat cream.

Nutrition:
- Calories: 776
- Fat: 56.8g
- Fiber: 0g
- Carbs: 58.5 g
- Protein: 14.2g
- Cholesterol 15mg
- Sodium 120mg

# Sweet Buns

Servings: 2    Prep time: 40min    Cook time: 30min

## INGREDIENTS

1/3 cup of psyllium husks
1/2 cup of coconut flour
2 tbsps of brown sugar
4 eggs
1 tsp of baking powder
1/2 tsp of cinnamon
1/2 tsp of cloves; ground
Some chocolate chips
1 cup of hot water
A pinch of salt

## DIRECTIONS

Mix flour with psyllium husks, brown sugar, baking powder, salt, cinnamon, cloves, and chocolate chips in a bowl and stir well. Add water and eggs; mix well until you obtain a dough. Shape 8 buns, and arrange them on a lined baking sheet. Introduce in the oven at 350F/176C and bake for 30 minutes.

Nutrition:
- Calories 599
- Fat: 16.9g
- Carbs: 130.5g
- Protein: 16.9g
- Cholesterol 330mg
- Sodium 557mg

# Rice Pudding

Servings: 2      Prep time: 5 min                    Cook time: 20 min

## INGREDIENTS

1-1/2 cups milk
1/4 cup long-grain rice
4 tbsps sugar
1/2 tsp salt
1/4 cup raisins
1 tsp vanilla extract
Ground cinnamon

## DIRECTIONS

In a saucepan, mix milk, rice, sugar, and salt; bring to a boil over medium heat, stirring constantly. Boil for 15 minutes; add raisins and vanilla and boil until rice is tender. Sprinkle with cinnamon and serve warm or refrigerate and serve cold.

Nutrition:
- Calories: 214
- Fat: 3g
- Fiber: 1g
- Carbs: 41 g
- Protein: 6g
- Cholesterol 11mg
- Sodium 266mg

# Cream Pie

Servings: 2      Prep time: 15 min                    Cook time: 15 min

## INGREDIENTS

1-3/4 cups graham cracker crumbs
1/4 cup sugar, divided
1/4 cup butter, melted
1/2 envelope of gelatin
4 tbsps cold water
1 cup of cream cheese
1 cup heavy whipping cream
1 tsp vanilla extract
Mixed fresh berries

Nutrition:
- Calories 1199
- Fat: 90.4g
- Carbs: 83.3g
- Protein: 18..6g
- Cholesterol 271mg
- Sodium 893mg

## DIRECTIONS

Preheat oven to 350F/176C. Combine cracker crumbs and half of the sugar with melted butter. Using the bottom of a glass, press the cracker mixture onto the bottom and up the sides of greased dish pie plate. Bake until set, 12 min. Cool completely. Sprinkle gelatin over cold water, and let stand for 5 min. Beat cream cheese and remaining sugar until smooth. Slowly beat in cream and vanilla. Microwave gelatin on high until melted, about 10 sec. Beat into cream cheese mixture. Transfer filling to crust. Refrigerate covered until set, about 3 hours. Top with mixed fresh berries.

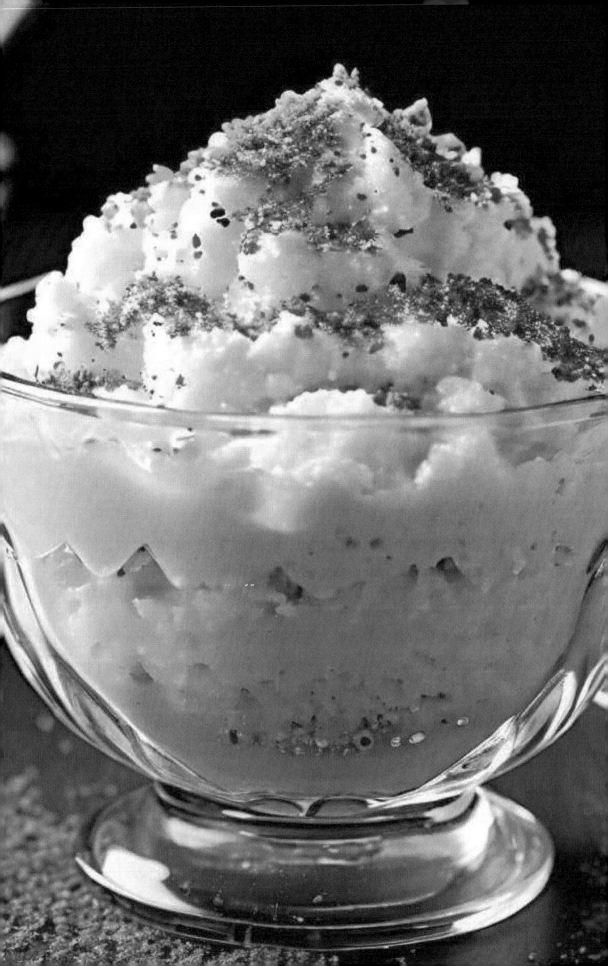

# Chocolate Mousse

Servings: 2      Prep time: 10min+2h      Cook time: 3min

## INGREDIENTS

1/4 cup chocolate chips

1 tbsp water

1 large egg yolk, lightly beaten

1-1/2 tsps vanilla extract

1/2 cup heavy whipping cream

1 tbsp sugar

Nutrition:
- Calories: 367
- Fat: 13g
- Fiber: 1g
- Carbs: 21 g
- Protein: 3g
- Cholesterol 188mg
- Sodium 29mg

## DIRECTIONS

In a small saucepan, melt chocolate chips with water; stir until smooth. Stir a small amount of hot chocolate mixture into egg yolk; return all to the pan, stirring constantly. Cook and stir for 2 minutes or until slightly thickened. Remove from the heat; stir in vanilla. Quickly transfer to a small bowl. Stir occasionally until completely cooled. In a small bowl, beat whipping cream until it begins to thicken. Add sugar; beat until soft peaks form. Fold into cooled chocolate mixture. Cover and refrigerate for at least 2 hours.

# Shortbread Cookies

Servings: 2      Prep time: 15min      Cook time: 30min

## INGREDIENTS

1 cup unsalted butter, softened

1/2 cup sugar

2 cups all-purpose flour

Confectioners' sugar

Nutrition 1 cookie:
- Calories: 183
- Fat: 12 g
- Carbs: 18g
- Protein: 2g
- Cholesterol: 31mg
- Sodium: 2mg

## DIRECTIONS

Preheat oven to 360F/180C. Cream butter and sugar until light and fluffy. Gradually beat in flour. Press dough into an ungreased 9-inch. square baking pan. Prick with a fork. Bake until light brown, 30-35 minutes. Cut into 16 squares while warm. Cool completely on a wire rack. Dust with confectioners' sugar.

# Apple Cake

Servings: 2      Prep time:10min                    Cook time:55min

## INGREDIENTS

2 cups all-purpose flour, divided

1/4 tsp salt

1/2 cups cold butter, divided

3 to 4 tbsps ice water

5 cups thinly sliced peeled tart apples (about 8 medium)

1/2 cup sugar, divided

2 tsps ground cinnamon

Nutrition:
- Calories: 1187
- Fat: 47.7g
- Fiber: 8.2g
- Carbs: 182.4g
- Protein: 14.2g
- Cholesterol 122mg
- Sodium 621mg

## DIRECTIONS

Preheat oven to 360F/180C. Mix 2 cups of flour with salt and 1 cup of butter. Add ice water to form moist crumbs. Press the mixture onto the bottom of a greased baking pan. Bake until lightly browned, 20 min. Cool on the wire rack. In a large bowl, combine apples, 1 cup of sugar, and cinnamon and toss to coat. Spoon over the crust. Mix remaining flour, butter, and sugar until coarse crumbs form. Sprinkle over apples. Bake until golden brown, and the apples are tender 40 min. Cool completely on a wire rack.

# Coffee Cake

Servings: 2      Prep time:15min                    Cook time:20min

## INGREDIENTS

1 cup self-raising flour

2 eggs

2 tbsp butter melted

2 tbsp coffee essence

1/4 cup sugar

2 tbs milk cold

## DIRECTIONS

Mix eggs yolks with sugar until it is fluffy and 3 x volume. Mix eggs white separately until solid. Mix melted butter, flour, sugar, and milk until smooth. Add white eggs and mix with a spatula. Bake for 20 min at 360F/180C, or until baked, test with a skewer.

Nutrition:
- Calories 528
- Fat: 17g
- Carbs: 82.1g
- Protein: 12.8g
- Cholesterol 196mg
- Sodium 70mg

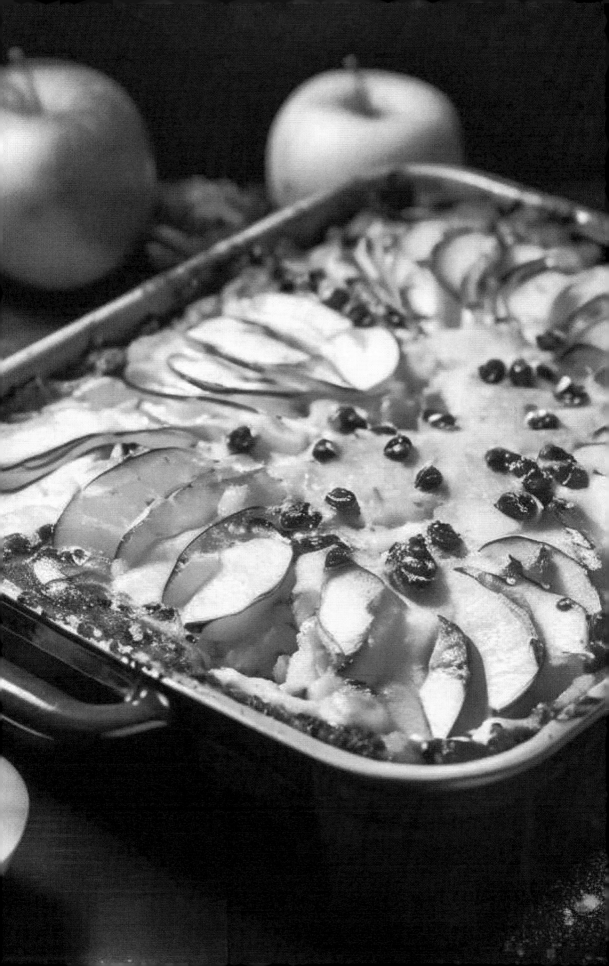

# Chip Cookies

Servings: 2    Prep time:15min              Cook time:11min

## INGREDIENTS

1/2 cup butter, softened

1/4 cup sugar

1/4 cup packed brown sugar

2 large eggs

1 tbs vanilla extract

1-1/2 cups all-purpose flour

1 tbs baking soda

  pinch salt

1/2 cup dried cranberries

1/2 cup chopped pecans

Nutrition:
- Calories: 1244
- Fat: 86.5g
- Fiber: 7.9g
- Carbs: 101.2g
- Protein: 18.5g
- Cholesterol 308mg
- Sodium 2369mg

## DIRECTIONS

Preheat oven to 375F/190C. In a large bowl, cream butter and sugars until light and fluffy. Add eggs, one at a time, beating well after each addition. Add in vanilla. Combine the flour, baking soda, and salt; gradually add to the creamed mixture and mix well. Stir in the cranberries and pecans. Drop by tablespoonfuls apart onto ungreased baking sheets. Bake until golden brown, 9-11 minutes. Cool on pans for 2 minutes before removing to wire racks to cool completely.

# Banana Bread

Servings: 2    Prep time:15min              Cook time:35min

## INGREDIENTS

1-1/2 cups all-purpose flour

1 teaspoon baking soda

1 cup brown sugar

1/2 cup water

1/3 cup mashed ripe bananas
(about 1 small)

1/4 cup canola oil

1/2 teaspoon vanilla extract

## DIRECTIONS

Preheat oven to 350F/176C. In a bowl, combine flour and baking soda. Whisk brown sugar, water, banana, oil, and vanilla in another bowl. Stir into dry ingredients just until moistened. Transfer to a greased baking pan. Bake until a toothpick inserted in the center comes out clean, 30-35 minutes. Cool on a wire rack. Cut into 9 pieces.

Nutrition:
- Calories 792
- Fat: 28g
- Carbs: 130.5g
- Protein: 7.1g
- Cholesterol 0mg
- Sodium 653mg

# Oatmeal Bars with Dates

Servings: 2    Prep time:10min              Cook time:30min

## INGREDIENTS

1 cup pitted dates, quartered
3/4 cup water
1/4 cup sugar
3/4 cup all-purpose flour
3/4 cup old-fashioned oats
1 tsp vanilla extract
1/2 tsp baking soda
pinch salt
1/4 tsp almond extract
1/4 cup shortening

Nutrition:
- Calories: 804
- Fat: 27.6g
- Fiber: 9.9g
- Carbs: 138g
- Protein: 8.9g
- Cholesterol 0mg
- Sodium 398mg

## DIRECTIONS

Preheat oven to 350F/176C. In a saucepan, combine dates, water, and sugar, boil, simmer, uncovered, until thickened and dates are tender, stirring constantly, 7-9 minutes. Remove from heat. Combine flour, oats, vanilla, baking soda, salt, and almond extract in a bowl. Cut in shortening until crumbly. Press half onto the bottom of a greased baking dish. Carefully spread with date mixture. Sprinkle the remaining crumb mixture over the filling; press down gently. Bake until lightly browned, 25-30 minutes. Cool on a wire rack.

# Oat Bars

Servings: 2    Prep time:15min              Cook time:40min

## INGREDIENTS

1/4 cup raisins
3/4 cups boiling water
1 cup oats
1/4 cup packed brown sugar
1/4 cup milk
1 medium apple,
peeled and finely chopped
2 tablespoons butter, melted
1/4 cup chopped walnuts

## DIRECTIONS

Place raisins in a small bowl. Cover with boiling water; let stand for 5 minutes. Meanwhile, in a large bowl, combine the oats, brown sugar, milk, apple, and butter. Let stand for 5 minutes. Drain raisins; stir into oat mixture. Transfer to a baking dish coated with baking paper. Sprinkle with walnuts. Bake at 350F/176C for 30-35 minutes or until a knife inserted in the center comes out clean.

Nutrition:
- Calories 550
- Fat: 24.3 g
- Carbs: 78.3g
- Protein: 11.1g
- Cholesterol 33mg
- Sodium 110mg

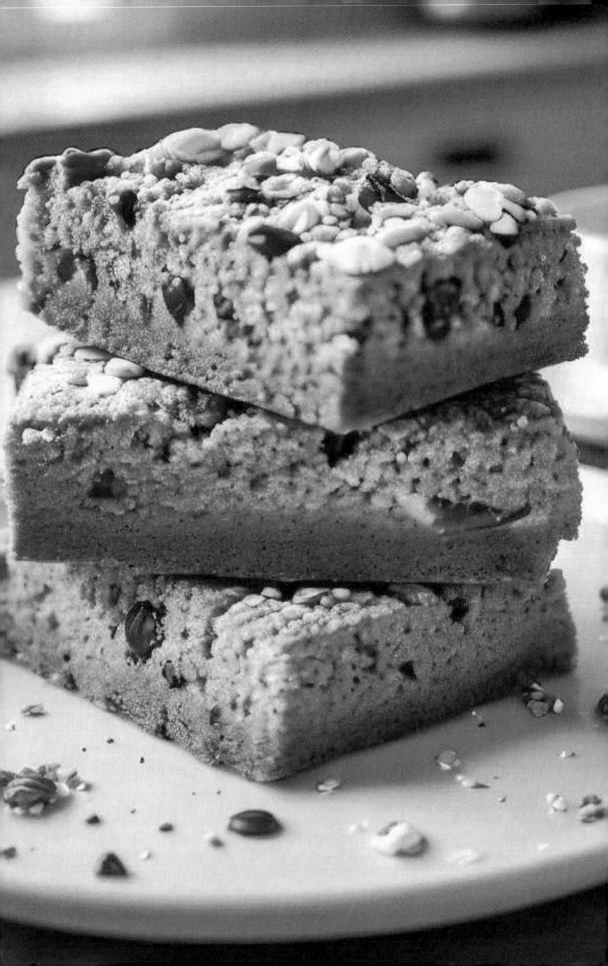

# DRESSING
# AND SAUCES

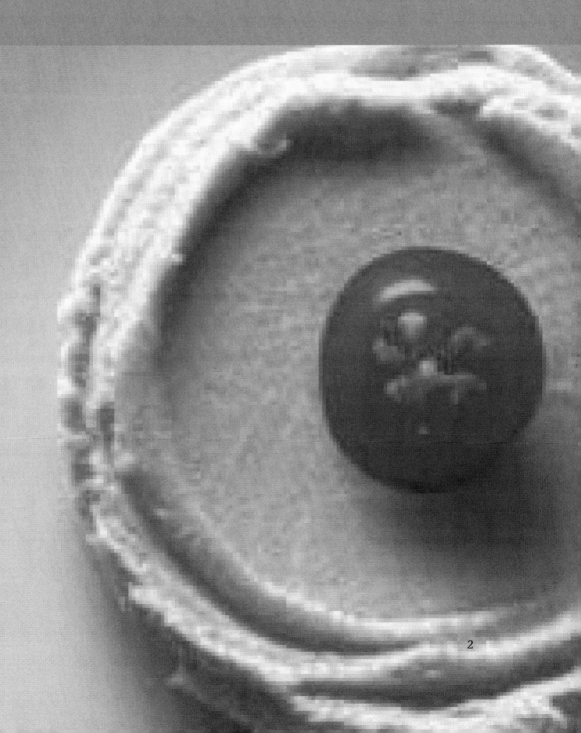

# Greek Yogurt Dressing

Servings: 2     Prep time: 10min     Cook time: 0min

## INGREDIENTS

1/2 cup Greek yogurt
2 tbsps lemon juice
1 tbsps extra virgin olive oil
1 clove garlic, minced
1 tbsps chopped fresh dill (or other herbs of your choice)
Salt and pepper to taste

## DIRECTIONS

In a small bowl, whisk together the Greek yogurt, lemon juice, olive oil, minced garlic, chopped dill, salt, and pepper until well combined. Adjust the seasoning according to your taste preferences. Drizzle the Greek yogurt dressing over your salad and toss well to coat.

Nutrition:
- Calories: 170
- Fat: 7.2g
- Fiber: 0.3g
- Carbs: 9.2g
- Protein: 19.3g
- Cholesterol 0mg
- Sodium 82mg

# Hummus

Servings: 2     Prep time: 15min     Cook time: 0min

## INGREDIENTS

1 can (15 ounces) chickpeas, drained and rinsed
3 tbsps tahini paste
2 tbsps lemon juice
2 cloves garlic, minced
2 tbsps extra virgin olive oil
1/2 tsp ground cumin
Salt and pepper to taste
Water (as needed)

## DIRECTIONS

Combine chickpeas, tahini paste, lemon juice, minced garlic, olive oil, cumin, salt, and pepper in a food processor or blender. Blend until smooth, adding water gradually to reach your desired consistency. Adjust the seasoning according to your taste preferences. Serve the hummus as a dip or use it as a salad or sandwich dressing.

Nutrition:
- Calories 407
- Fat: 4g
- Carbs: 33.5g
- Protein: 10.2g
- Cholesterol 0mg
- Sodium 389mg

# Classic Vinaigrette

Servings: 2    Prep time:10min         Cook time:0min

## INGREDIENTS

1/4 cup extra virgin olive oil
2 tbsps balsamic vinegar (or
any vinegar of your choice)
1 tsp Dijon mustard
1 clove garlic, minced
Salt and pepper to taste

## DIRECTIONS

Whisk together the olive oil, vinegar, Dijon mustard, minced garlic, salt, and pepper in a small bowl until well combined. Adjust the seasoning according to your taste preferences. Drizzle the vinaigrette over your salad and toss well to coat.

Nutrition:
- Calories: 223
- Fat: 25.3g
- Fiber: 0.1g
- Carbs: 0.8g
- Protein: 0.2g
- Cholesterol 0mg
- Sodium 29mg

# Tahini

Servings: 2         Prep time:15min       Cook time:0min

## INGREDIENTS

1 cup of sesame seeds
Salt and pepper to taste
3-4 tbsps olive oil

## DIRECTIONS

Throw sesame seeds into a vast, dry saucepan over medium-low heat, then stir constantly with a spoon until the seeds darken ever so slightly in color and become fragrant. Let them cold. Put them in a food processor or blender and blend until smooth. Add olive oil and blend until you get a paste. Put in a glass jar and keep in the refrigerator for a month. Use for Hummus or spread in the sandwich or as a dipping sauce.

Nutrition:
- Calories 593
- Fat: 56.8g
- Carbs: 16.9g
- Protein: 12.8g
- Cholesterol 0mg
- Sodium 8mg

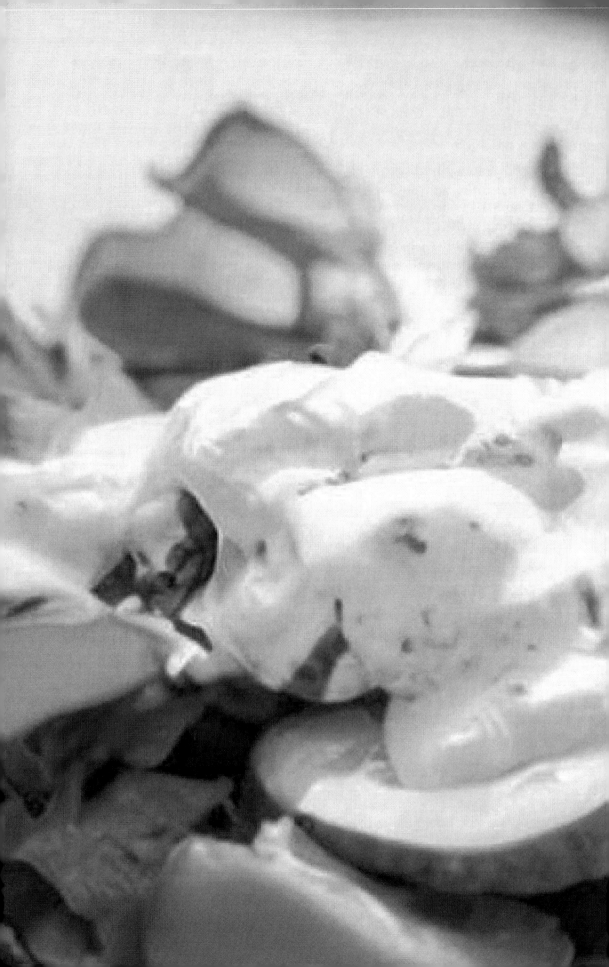

# Mustard

Servings: 2     Prep time:15min            Cook time:0min

## INGREDIENTS

6 tbsps mustard seeds
1/2 cup mustard powder
1/2 cup water
3 tbsps vinegar
1 tsp salt
1 tsp ground turmeric
1 tbsp honey - optional
1/4 cup minced fresh herbs
(like: parsley, fennel,
dill,chervil) - optional

Nutrition:
- Calories: 209
- Fat: 9.9g
- Fiber: 6.9g
- Carbs: 23.9g
- Protein: 9.1g
- Cholesterol 0mg
- Sodium 1170mg

## DIRECTIONS

Grind the whole mustard seeds in a spice or coffee grinder for a few seconds. Pour the semi-ground seeds into a bowl and add the salt and mustard powder. If using, add the optional ingredients, too. Pour in the water, then stir well. When everything is incorporated, let this sit for up to 10 minutes. When ready, pour in the vinegar. Pour into a glass jar and store in the fridge. It will be runny at first. Wait at least 12 hours before using it. It will last a year in the refrigerator.

# Tahini Dressing

Servings: 2     Prep time:15min            Cook time:0min

## INGREDIENTS

1/4 cup tahini paste

2 tbsps lemon juice

2 tbsps water

1 clove garlic, minced

1 tbsp extra virgin olive oil

Salt to taste

## DIRECTIONS

Whisk together the tahini paste, lemon juice, water, minced garlic, olive oil, and salt until smooth and creamy in a small bowl. If the dressing is too thick, add more water, one tablespoon at a time, until you reach the desired consistency. Drizzle the tahini dressing over your salad and toss well to coat.

Nutrition:
- Calories 244
- Fat: 23.3g
- Carbs: 7.2g
- Protein: 5.3g
- Cholesterol 0mg
- Sodium 116mg

# Mustard Dressing

### INGREDIENTS

1/4 cup extra virgin olive oil
2 tbsps mustard
2 tbsps lemon juice
1 tbsps honey (optional)
Salt and pepper to taste

### DIRECTIONS

In a small bowl, whisk together the olive oil, mustard, lemon juice, honey (if using), salt, and pepper until well combined. Adjust the seasoning according to your taste preferences. Drizzle the mustard dressing over your salad and toss well to coat.

Nutrition:
- Calories: 304
- Fat: 28.5g
- Fiber: 1.7g
- Carbs: 12.9g
- Protein: 3g
- Cholesterol 0mg
- Sodium 4mg

# Grill Sauce

### INGREDIENTS

1 bunch parsley, stems removed
½ cup fresh cilantro leaves
1/4 cup olive oil
¼ cup fresh oregano leaves
4 cloves garlic, chopped
3 tbsps white vinegar
¼ tsp ground cumin
¼ tsp red pepper flakes
black pepper, salt

### DIRECTIONS

Combine all ingredients in a blender and blend until a thick sauce forms. This sauce is excellent on all kinds of grilled meats and fish.

Nutrition:
- Calories 487
- Fat: 51.7g
- Carbs: 10.3g
- Protein: 2.4g
- Cholesterol 0mg
- Sodium 23mg

# Hot Mango Sauce

Servings: 2    Prep time:15min        Cook time:0min

INGREDIENTS

¾ cup minced mango
¼ cup vinegar
juice from one lime
½ small Thai chile pepper, minced
1 clove garlic, crushed
1 tbs hot chile paste
1 tbsp chopped fresh cilantro

DIRECTIONS

Stir all ingredients in a bowl until well combined. Cover and let rest for 30 min. Use with grilled meat or fish.

Nutrition:
- Calories: 56
- Fat: 0.3g
- Fiber: 1.5g
- Carbs: 13g
- Protein: 0.9g
- Cholesterol 0mg
- Sodium 4mg

# Fresh Sauce

Servings: 2        Prep time:15min        Cook time:0min

INGREDIENTS

1/4 cup greek yoghurt
1/4 cup hummus
1/2 cup cornichons, finely chopped
½ bunch fresh dill, finely chopped
2 tbsps capers, chopped
1 medium lemon, juiced
1 tsp mustard
1 small clove garlic, minced
1 pinch cayenne pepper, or more to taste

DIRECTIONS

Stir all ingredients in a bowl. This sauce is excellent on all kinds of fish.

Nutrition:
- Calories 107
- Fat: 6.2g
- Carbs: 11.6g
- Protein: 5.5g
- Cholesterol 0mg
- Sodium 976mg

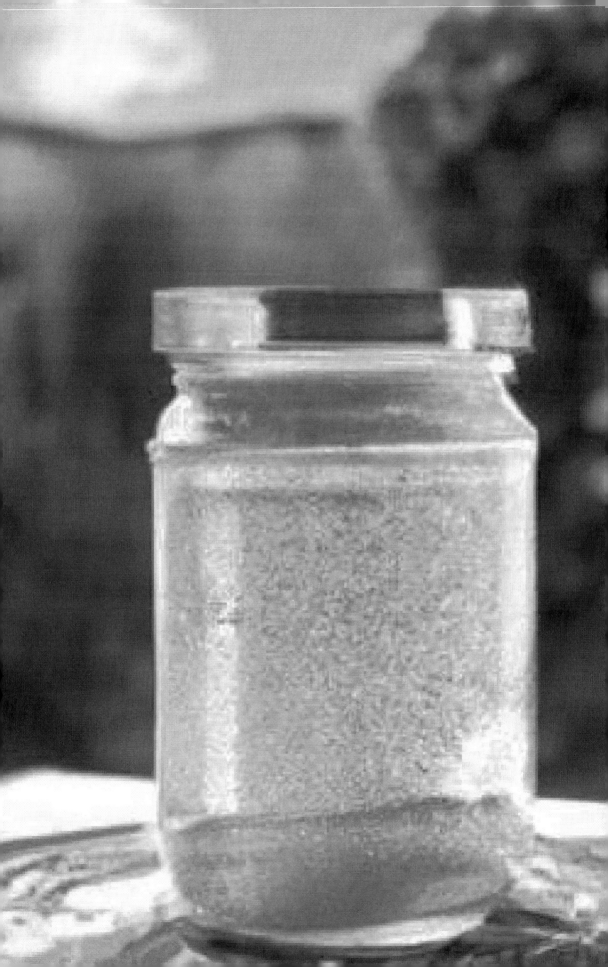

# Lemon and Caper Dressing

Servings: 2    Prep time:10min          Cook time:0min

## INGREDIENTS

1 garlic clove
1/4 tsp Black pepper
1 tbsp capers (about 18)
3 tbsp freshly squeezed lemon juice
2 tbsp grated Parmesan
¼ cup olive oil

## DIRECTIONS

Coarsely mince the garlic. Add fresh pepper and the capers to the garlic. Chop and press down on the mixture with the side of your knife until a paste forms. Put the paste into a bowl and add the lemon juice and Parmesan. Slowly add in the olive oil, stirring until emulsified.

Use it or keep it covered for up to 2 days in the fridge. Good with grilled vegetables.

Nutrition:
- Calories: 315
- Fat: 31g
- Fiber: 0.3g
- Carbs: 24g
- Protein: 9.4g
- Cholesterol 20mg
- Sodium 392mg

# Pomegranate Dressing

Servings: 2          Prep time:15min          Cook time:0min

## INGREDIENTS

2 tbsp pomegranate juice (or make juice from seeds of ½ pomegranate)
2 tbsp extra-virgin olive oil
1 tbsp white wine vinegar
seeds from 1/2 pomegranate
1/4 tsp caster sugar

## DIRECTIONS

Combine all the ingredients in a bowl, and stir well. Use as a dressing for couscous, rice, or green salad. Keep it in the fridge for up to 5 days.

Nutrition:
- Calories 124
- Fat: 14g
- Carbs: 0.7g
- Protein: 0g
- Cholesterol 0mg
- Sodium 0mg

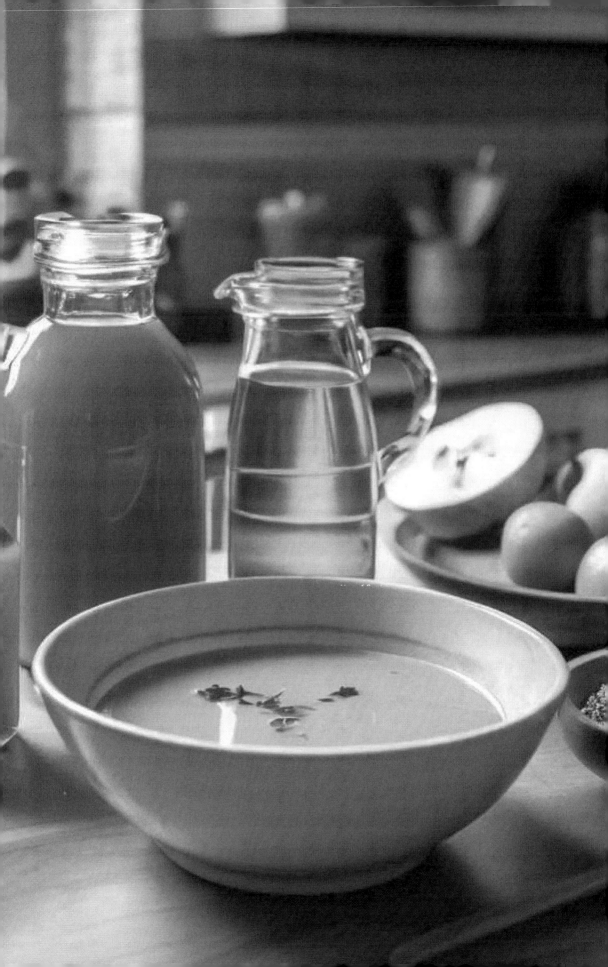

# Spice Sauce

Servings: 2    Prep time:15min        Cook time:0min

## INGREDIENTS

2 tbsp hot chili sauce
1 tbsp soy sauce
1 tbsp honey or brown sugar
1 tsp minced garlic
1 tsp grated ginger
1 tbsp lime juice
1 tbsp olive oil
Salt and pepper

Nutrition:
- Calories:109
- Fat: 7.1g
- Fiber: 0.4g
- Carbs: 12.5g
- Protein: 0.9g
- Cholesterol 0mg
- Sodium 833mg

## DIRECTIONS

In a small bowl, combine the hot chili sauce, soy sauce, honey or brown sugar, minced garlic, grated ginger, lime juice, salt, pepper, and olive oil. Mix the ingredients well until the sauce is smooth and all the flavors are incorporated.

Once the sauce is ready, you can use it immediately or refrigerate it briefly to allow the flavors to meld. When grilling the beef or fish, brush a thin layer of the spicy chili sauce onto the meat before placing it on the grill.

# Basil Pesto

Servings: 2    Prep time:15min        Cook time:0min

## INGREDIENTS

2 cups fresh basil leaves
1/3 cup walnuts, toasted
1/4 cup grated Parmesan cheese
1 clove garlic
1/4 cup extra-virgin olive oil
1 teaspoon lemon juice
Salt and pepper

Nutrition:
- Calories 533
- Fat: 49.7g
- Carbs: 5.3g
- Protein: 23.9g
- Cholesterol 40mg
- Sodium 522mg

## DIRECTIONS

In a food processor, combine the toasted walnuts, fresh basil leaves, garlic, and grated Parmesan cheese. Pulse the mixture a few times until the ingredients are coarsely chopped. With the food processor running, slowly drizzle in the extra-virgin olive oil until the mixture becomes a smooth and creamy consistency. Add the lemon juice and a pinch of salt and pepper. Blend again to incorporate the flavors. Good with cooked pasta, as a topping for grilled vegetables, or as a spread on whole-grain toast.

# Ginger Turmeric

## INGREDIENTS

1/4 cup olive oil

2 tbsp apple cider vinegar

1 tsp turmeric

1/2 tsp ground ginger

## DIRECTIONS

Stir all ingredients in a bowl. This sauce is excellent for bean salads, mixed greens, or veggie bowls.

Nutrition:
- Calories 225
- Fat: 25.2g
- Carbs: 1.2g
- Protein: 0.1g
- Cholesterol 0mg
- Sodium 1mg

# INDEX

# Index in Alphabetical Order

Dear Reader,

I hope you enjoyed the book and that it has brought you closer to achieving your goals. Your journey and growth as a reader mean a lot to me, and I genuinely hope this book has played a significant role in helping you along the way.

I wanted to ask if you would be open to leaving a review on Amazon. I understand if you'd prefer not to, as your time is valuable. However, your review would be incredibly valuable to me, as it would help me understand what my readers appreciate and what they don't. I assure you that I read all of the reviews and carefully consider them when writing the next book. Simply share a few words about your thoughts.

Thank you for considering this request, and please know that I sincerely appreciate your support.

Wishing you continued success and all the best,

Danielle De Mayo

danielledemayoo@gmail.com

Made in the USA
Las Vegas, NV
10 May 2024

89769176R00105